AN INTRODUCTION TO FUNCTIONAL OCCLUSION

MAJOR M. ASH, B.S., D.D.S., M.S.

Professor and Chairman
Department of Occlusion
School of Dentistry
University of Michigan
Ann Arbor, Michigan

SIGURD P. RAMFJORD, L.D.S., Ph.D.

Professor of Dentistry
School of Dentistry
University of Michigan
Ann Arbor, Michigan

1982

W. B. SAUNDERS COMPANY
Philadelphia   London   Toronto   Sydney   Tokyo   Mexico City

W. B. Saunders Company: West Washington Square
Philadelphia, PA 19105

1 St. Anne's Road
Eastbourne, East Sussex BN21 3UN, England

1 Goldthorne Avenue
Toronto, Ontario M8Z 5T9, Canada

9 Waltham Street
Artarmon, N.S.W. 2064, Australia

Library of Congress Cataloging in Publication Data

Ash, Major M.

An introduction to functional occlusion.

1. Dental articulators.   2. Occlusion (Dentistry)   3. Splints,
Bite plane.   I. Ramfjord, Sigurd Peder, 1911–   II. Title.
[DNLM: 1. Dental equipment.   2. Dental occlusion.
WU 440 A819i]

RK685.A75A83   617.6'43   81–5275

ISBN 0–7216–1428–0   AACR2

An Introduction to Functional Occlusion   ISBN   0-7216-1428-0

Last digit is the print number: 9   8   7   6   5   4   3

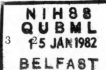

Contributors

JOSEPH A. CLAYTON, D.D.S., M.S.
Professor of Dentistry
Department of Crown and Bridge
School of Dentistry
The University of Michigan
Ann Arbor, Michigan

WALTER KOVALESKI, III, D.D.S.,
M.S.
Associate Professor of Dentistry
Department of Occlusion
School of Dentistry
The University of Michigan
Ann Arbor, Michigan

SALLY HOLDEN, R.D.H., R.D.A.,
M.S.
Associate Professor of Dental Hygiene
School of Dentistry
The University of Michigan
Ann Arbor, Michigan

CHARLES B. CARTWRIGHT, D.D.S.,
M.S.
Professor of Dentistry
Assistant Dean, Postgraduate Dentistry
School of Dentistry
The University of Michigan
Ann Arbor, Michigan

E. RICHARD McPHEE, D.D.S., M.S.
Professor of Dentistry
Department of Crown and Bridge
School of Dentistry
The University of Michigan
Ann Arbor, Michigan

HARVEY W. SCHIELD, D.D.S., M.S.
Professor of Dentistry
Director of PreClinical Dentistry
School of Dentistry
The University of Michigan
Ann Arbor, Michigan

GEORGE M. ASH, D.D.S., M.S.
Assistant Professor
PreClinical Dentistry
School of Dentistry
The University of Michigan
Ann Arbor, Michigan

JEFFREY L. ASH, D.D.S., M.S.
Assistant Professor
Department of Endodontics
School of Dentistry
The University of Michigan
Ann Arbor, Michigan

WILLIAM KOTOWICZ, D.D.S., M.S.
Professor of Dentistry
Partial Denture Department
School of Dentistry
The University of Michigan
Ann Arbor, Michigan

RICHARD A. REED, D.D.S., M.S.
Associate Professor of Dentistry
Department of Occlusion
School of Dentistry
The University of Michigan
Ann Arbor, Michigan

Preface

It has become apparent that the application of some of the principles of current concepts of occlusion would be enhanced if the details of several of the clinical and technical procedures were made available in the form of a manual. Because of the nature of these details of procedure, only a few aspects of theory will be provided in this manual, and the reader is referred to selected references for additional sources of information.

The basic elements for the use of an articulator, the waxing of restorations, and the waxing of an occlusal bite plane splint are provided for the student in the literature. The utilization of a Hanau H2–PR articulator is not an endorsement of this articulator; many other types of semi-adjustable articulators (Denar, Whip–Mix, Condylator, Dentatus, etc.) may also be used.

The contents of this manual have been used in teaching undergraduate and graduate students for more than two decades. Although several aspects may be directed toward the concept of "freedom in centric," the primary goals relate to enlightened use of an articulator and prevention of occlusal dysfunction through functional or diagnostic waxing of restorations or through both. Some concepts presented here have been outlined in *Functional Occlusion I* and *II*, workbooks produced jointly by the Department of Occlusion and the Department of Educational Resources of the University of Michigan School of Dentistry. In this respect we wish to acknowledge the assistance of Dr. Dave Starks, Chairman of the Department of Educational Resources, and Terisita M. Tchou, B.S.E., M.A., Senior Instructional Associate.

Although this manual reflects concepts taught by us for more than 25 years in our courses on occlusion, and even though it would be difficult if not impossible to describe the contribution made by individual teachers, we wish to acknowledge their contributions to the development of the material used in our courses.

We wish to thank Professor William Brudon for many of the illustrations characterized by his excellent appreciation for form and function. We acknowledge also the contributions made by Dr. Jose dos Santos, Dr. James O. Bailey, and by Ms. Karen Smith.

For the excellent photographic services we wish to acknowledge Mike Kvicala, Keary Campbell and Per Kjeldson. The assistance of Mrs. Marian Brockie and Mrs. Norma Staples in the preparation of the manuscript has been invaluable, and is gratefully acknowledged.

Several television tapes have been developed for the subject matter of this manual by Drs. Robert Brodbelt, Christian Stohler, Terrance Timm, and Joseph Clayton. Inquiries regarding these TV productions may be directed to the Department of Occlusion, The University of Michigan, School of Dentistry, Ann Arbor, Michigan, 48103.

MAJOR M. ASH, JR.
SIGURD P. RAMFJORD

Contents

Unit 1

Concepts of Occlusion

The term "occlusion" is usually defined in relation to contacting surfaces of the teeth, but the conceptual view should include all the functional, parafunctional, and dysfunctional relationships that exist between the components of the masticatory system as a result of the contacts between the occlusal surfaces of the teeth. In this sense "occlusion" is defined as the functional and dysfunctional relationships between an integrated system of teeth, supporting structures, joints, and neuromuscular components. The definition includes psychological as well as physiological aspects of function and dysfunction.

INTRODUCTION: UNIT OBJECTIVES AND READINGS

The objectives for this unit are to present some of the concepts of occlusion that are necessary for the application of the principles of occlusion to clinical practice, and for an understanding of the other units in this manual.

A. Objectives
1. Be able to define:
   a. Functional occlusion
   b. Centric occlusion
   c. Centric relation
   d. Freedom in centric
   e. Bennett movement
   f. "Normal" occlusion
   g. Terminal hinge axis
   h. Vertical dimension
   i. Slide in centric
   j. Guidance
   k. Curve of Spee
   l. Balanced occlusion

2. Be able to describe:
   a. Border movements of the mandible in the sagittal and horizontal planes
   b. Movement paths made by the supporting cusps of first molars
   c. Centric stops for all supporting cusps for all teeth.
3. Be able to relate the determinants of occlusion with occlusal morphology.
4. Be able to outline the requirements for transfer of information from the patient to an articulator.

B. Reading (optional)
Ramfjord, S. O., and Ash, M. M., Jr.: Occlusion. Philadelphia, W. B. Saunders Co., 1971, Chapters 4 and 10.

UNIFIED CONCEPT OF OCCLUSION

A number of approaches to occlusion have been suggested, but only the concept of "freedom in centric" is complete and open for all areas of dental practice. A system of ideas that may be put to practical use, and which can be understood as a unified concept of occlusion, is necessary for effective treatment of patients. In order to aid in promoting or developing a functional occlusion, or in preventing dysfunctional occlusion, the concept must be flexible enough to be applied to the wide variety of occlusal problems that exist in clinical dentistry. The system of ideas expressed here provides the practical basis for a concept of functional occlusion consistent with the principles of occlusion relevant to the practice of dentistry.

A *practical concept of occlusion* must be open-ended — that is, useful for restorative dentistry, orthodontics, treatment of functional disturbances, and for individual teeth as well as full mouth reconstruction. It should not be closed to individual restorations or to any type of dental practice, or be limited by economics. A *complete concept of occlusion* should include rational and practical ideas that are biologically acceptable on centric occlusion, centric relation, vertical dimension, rest position, mandibular guidance, and occlusal stability. The relationship between the total masticatory system and the individual—including the relationship between occlusion, swallowing, mastication, and parafunction — should be considered.

FUNCTIONAL OCCLUSION: DEFINITION AND SCOPE

The term *functional occlusion* means conducive to function and refers to a state of the occlusion: (1) in which the occlusal interfaces are free of interferences to smooth gliding movements of the mandible, (2) there is freedom for the mandible to close or to be guided into maximum intercuspation in centric occlusion and centric relation, and (3) in which occlusal contact relations contribute to occlusal stability.

From a practical standpoint functional occlusion refers to a state of harmonious function obtainable by an occlusal adjustment or by properly designed individual or multiple restorations or by both adjustment and restorations. Although orthodontics could be added as well, it will not be considered here. From previous reading, the reader should already be familiar with the terms *normal occlusion* and *ideal occlusion*. The term *ideal occlusion* is a conceptual goal for an ideal occlusal state; it is not constrained by the limitations of treatment. An occlusion may be functional without being entirely esthetic. Also, a functional occlusion may be developed for only parts of the occlusal interface by occlusal adjustment and properly waxed or carved restorations, yet some residual need for adaptation will remain because total treatment to reach an ideal occlusion cannot be or is not accomplished.

The way the teeth come together or occlude in function (mastication, swallowing, and so forth) is important for the health and comfort of the masticatory system. Restoring the teeth with inlays, crowns, or other restorations with occlusal surfaces that are conducive to optimal contact relations is a primary goal of restorative dentistry.

The objectives of this manual are to present practical methods for establishing functional occlusal contact relations for teeth or parts of teeth that have been lost because of disease. When the contacting surfaces of the occluding teeth (also called the *occlusal interfaces*) have functional rather than dysfunctional contact relations, the occlusion is considered to be functional.

The development of a functional occlusion for individual or multiple restorations in many instances requires that the restorations be made away from the patient. Hence the need for a simulator of the patient's jaws, teeth, and jaw movements. The simulation is done with an *articulator*, in which casts of the patient's dental arches are brought together (articulated) in functional positions. In order to have the teeth occlude in an articulator in the same way as in the patient, the articulator must be close to the same size as the patient's jaws and have elements that simulate the temporomandibular joints. It must also be capable of being adjusted to allow the teeth of the casts to come together as in the mouth. The size of the articulator is important because the mandible rotates and translates about the temporomandibular joints, and the same sized arcs of closure cannot be duplicated on a small articulator.

In order to position casts in an articulator so that the arcs of closure are the same as in the mouth, it is necessary to transfer the position of the maxillary arch relative to the condyles to the articulator. The mounting of the mandibular cast is related to the two positions, centric relation and centric occlusion. When properly mounted on the articulator, the casts should be able to occlude as the teeth do in the mouth, i.e., in centric relation and centric occlusion, as well as in lateral and protrusive excursions.

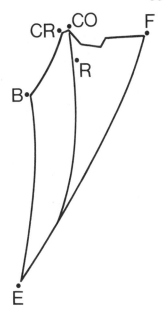

Figure 1–1. Envelope of border movements (sagittal plane). *CR*, centric relation; *CO*, centric occlusion; *B*, opening to maximum on the hinge axis; *E*, maximum opening; *R*, rest position; *F*, maximum protrusion.

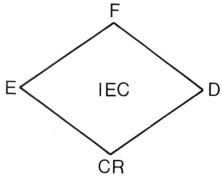

Figure 1–2. Envelope of border movements (horizontal plane). *CR*, centric relation; *E*, left lateral; *F*, protrusive; *D*, right lateral movement path; *IEC*, incisal edge contact.

JAW POSITIONS AND MOVEMENTS

Only a few mandibular positions are usually described in studying functional occlusion: centric occlusion, centric relation, and rest position in the sagittal plane; and working (functional) and balancing (nonfunctional) sides in the horizontal or frontal planes. Condylar positions may also be described as working (rotating) and balancing (orbiting) sides.

Border Movements

Movements of the mandible are very complex and difficult to describe. However, all jaw movements take place within certain boundaries. These boundaries constitute an envelope shown for the sagittal plane in Figure 1–1. Such an envelope can be envisioned as resulting from following a point on an incisor. Some of the earliest research done on mandibular movements was accomplished using a very small light attached to the incisors and exposing a photographic plate in a darkroom during mandibular movements. If a pencil were attached to the incisors during opening, closing, protrusive, and retrusive movements, an envelope of border movements would be produced as indicated in Figure 1–1. Centric occlusion and centric relation are on the sagittal plane envelope.

The envelope of border movements for

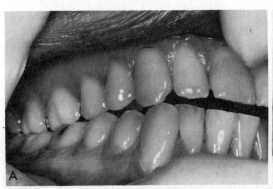
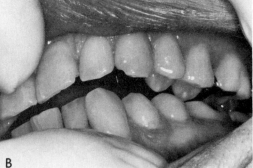

Figure 1–3. Border movements. *A*, right working (functional) side; *B*, left balancing (nonfunctional) side.

the horizontal plane is shown in Figure 1–2. This envelope not only contains functional contacts on the working side but extends well beyond masticatory function. Working side contact begins with lateral movement from maximum interdigitation outward to edge-to-edge contact of the buccal cusp tips. However, most function occurs within 1 to 2 mm of complete closure of the jaws. Working and balancing relations are demonstrated in Figure 1–3.

Movement Paths

Paths made by supporting cusps during mandibular movements can be superimposed over drawings of the teeth (Fig. 1–4). The paths are influenced by a number of factors such as intercondylar distance. These factors are summarized in this unit under the heading *Determinants of Occlusion.* Movement paths and their relationship to restorations and occlusal therapy must be envisioned for every supporting cusp. However, the relationship between mandibular movements and ridge and groove direction of the occlusal surfaces is not remarkable. Even so, it would not be appropriate to disregard potential sources of occlusal dysfunction.

Interferences

Interferences to closure into maximum intercuspation is referred to as a *premature*

contact in centric. A contact on the balancing side that causes disclusion of the teeth on the working side or displacement of a balancing side tooth is called a *balancing interference.* An occlusal contact on the working side that hampers smooth gliding occlusal contact movements on the working side is termed a *working interference.* A *protrusive interference* is an occlusal contact that causes disclusion of the anterior teeth or excessive movement of anterior teeth in protrusive movements. Any posterior contact in protrusive movements in the natural dentition is referred to as a protrusive interference except where anterior guidance is impossible, viz., anterior open bite. On mounted casts interferences can be judged only on the basis of disclusion effects and interference with smooth gliding movements.

Recordings of Mandibular Movements

Intraoral graphic registration of centric relation contact and posterior lateral border movements is sometimes used in dental procedures, especially in making complete dentures. The registration results in a "gothic arch" or "arrow point" tracing as seen in Figure 1–5. The stylus may be fixed to either the maxilla or the mandible (in this case, the maxilla). The stylus is set with a slight occlusal vertical opening so that the mandible may move freely without occlusal interference. The plate to be marked with the stylus is coated with dye, ink, wax, or other suitable material that can be scribed easily. On centric relation closure to contact, the stylus will make a mark at the apex of the gothic arch. The gothic arch tracing, pantograph, and other tracing devices are used to program or adjust an articulator so that casts of a patient mounted in the articulator more accurately simulate the patient's jaw movements, occlusal relationships, and jaw positions.

Condylar Movement

In addition to rotation and translation of the condyles during movement of the mandible, an immediate and progressive side shift of the condyle has been proposed. However, a side movement on the working side may be far less with the teeth in con-

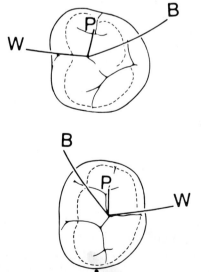

Figure 1–4. Movement paths. Paths made by supporting cusp on the right maxillary first molar (no. 3), and on the right mandibular first molar (no. 30). *W,* working; *P,* protrusive; *B,* balancing.

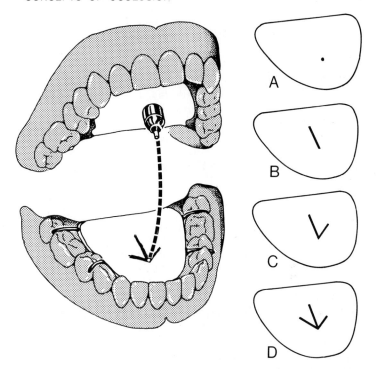

Figure 1–5. Gothic arch tracing. Smoked recording plate supported on lower teeth and intraoral stylus on the maxillary arch. *A*, centric relation; *B*, protrusive; *C*, right working added; *D*, left working added and completed gothic arch tracing.

tact than when there is no guidance. Although the exact lateral shift is difficult to determine, the incorporation of some side movement into an articulator takes little effort. Because of the potential benefit and the small expenditure of effort involved, it would seem appropriate to include the movement in the program of an articulator.

CENTRIC OCCLUSION

When the patient brings the teeth together so there is maximum intercuspation (centric occlusion), the number of contacts made by opposing teeth will be greater than if the patient is lightly bringing the jaws together without clenching or "biting hard." This difference in contacts can be demonstrated by placing thin (0.0005 in) plastic strips called *shim stock* between the occlusal surfaces and biting down with different amounts of muscle power. When an impression is made of a patient's teeth in order to make casts of stone or plaster, the teeth are not subjected to occlusal forces that occur when centric occlusion is obtained in the mouth by the patient. Thus the centric occlusion that can be obtained on casts is not the complete intercuspation that is obtained in the mouth. Such errors are not large but must be accounted for in the analysis of the occlusal contacts made for casts on the articulator.

Centric occlusion, also called the intercuspal position (IC), is probably the most important occlusal position of the teeth. It is the terminal position of the last stages of chewing and is frequently used as the position for bracing the mandible during swallowing. In some respects description of centric occlusion as a position is difficult, inasmuch as there are no measurements for precisely locating it to reference points in the jaws. Thus with the extraction of all the teeth centric occlusion is lost for the natural dentition. It is usually changed with comprehensive orthodontics. Even though centric occlusion cannot be precisely measured, it does have vertical and horizontal components. However, only the horizontal (lateral and anterior-posterior) components relative to centric relation can be measured for clinical purposes.

Centric occlusion may be considered as the terminal position of the open and close clench, of the closing chewing stroke, and of swallowing and yawning. However, such a terminal position is not actually centric occlusion by definition but could be if it were the same position that ensues with maximum intercuspation. Aside from a small error, the terminal position of the initial contact of an open and close clench is that position found in maximum intercuspation. The small positional difference between the terminal position of function and centric occlusion is dependent upon several variables. If centric occlusion is considered to be a position of the mandible and the teeth determined by three coordinates (a three-dimensional position), then a major variable could be the force of the "bite." "Maximum" intercuspation does not necessarily mean maximum force of bite, but there is some relationship between the degree of clench and the degree of intercuspation.

Another variable involves the status of the joints and muscles. With only a slight reservation centric occlusion can be related to centric stops on supporting cusps, fossae, and marginal ridges. The collective position of all these contact areas is related functionally to the positions of the condyles when the teeth are in maximal intercuspation. Any abnormality of the joints and muscles may interfere with the position of the condyles (vertically, laterally, and anterior-posteriorly) and prevent achievement of centric occlusion.

When a full gold crown restoration is made for a tooth such as a molar, it is cemented into place with a film of cement that is at best no thinner than 20 microns. Assuming that the centric occlusion positions for opposing teeth do not change as a result of the preparation of the tooth for restoration, the new contacts will be 20 microns too "high" in centric occlusion. If left unadjusted, the increased height may result in psychological responses inasmuch as many individuals can detect spaces of much less than 20 microns between the teeth. Some natural adjustment of function or structure or both may occur in response to the "high" restoration, but temporomandibular joint–muscle disturbances also may arise. Unless there is positional adaptation of the tooth with the high restoration, trauma from occlusion involving the periodontal structures can occur. Such changes can lead to a shifting of the teeth and centric occlusion. The use of inadequate temporary restorations may also cause a change in centric occlusion. Influences affecting centric occlusion include clenching, bruxism, wear, eruption, occlusal stability, loss of teeth, and restorations. When centric occlusion is lost as a point of reference for the masticatory system, the loss may result in physiological as well as psychological problems such as "phantom bite," i.e., multiple dysfunctional symptoms associated with the patient's

complaints of an inability to adjust to an alteration of centric occlusion.

When centric occlusion is changed or lost in a full mouth reconstruction, contact vertical dimension as well as the horizontal (lateral and anterior-posterior) components of centric occlusion must be approximated. An arbitrary vertical, lateral, or anterior-posterior placement of centric occlusion and hoped-for biological acceptance is all that is possible, because there is no scientific method of determining centric occlusion. On the basis of indirect evidence, it is assumed that all the factors mentioned can influence or change centric occlusion, but those factors contributing to occlusal stability tend to counteract such influences to maintain centric occlusion.

CENTRIC STOPS

The term *centric stop* refers to the occlusal contacts between supporting cusps and fossae or marginal ridges with the teeth in centric occlusion. The supporting cusps include the buccal cusps of the mandibular premolars and molars and the lingual cusps of maxillary premolars and molars. The cusps of the mandibular canines are supporting cusps and the mandibular incisors are treated as supporting cusps. Occlusal contacts between supporting cusps and fossae or marginal ridges can be related to what is considered to be an acceptable arrangement of the teeth, and the occlusion can be referred to as *Class I–normal*, using orthodontic terminology. It is a practical reference standard from which to describe an occlusion in terms of the position of teeth and centric stops (Fig. 1–6).

The presence, position, and morphological features of cusps, fossae, and marginal ridges that are centric stops significantly influence contact vertical dimension and occlusal stability. Failure to provide adequate centric stops can cause occlusal instability, resulting in shifting of the teeth and disturbances in muscles and joints. For example, centric stops should not be made in a restoration by placing a supporting cusp on a single inclined plane of a triangular cusp ridge. The contact relations for every supporting cusp must be visualized. For example, the distal buccal cusp of the mandibular first molar oc-

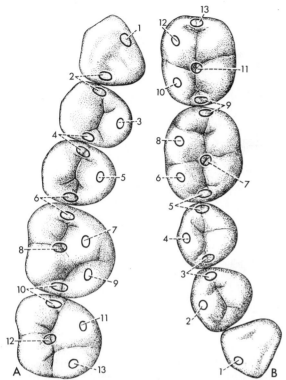

Figure 1–6. Centric stops. Position of centric stops in a normal (Angle class I) occlusion. Corresponding numbers on maxillary and mandibular teeth relate to contact of supporting cusps with fossae and marginal ridges of opposing teeth in centric occlusion.

cludes in the central fossa of the maxillary first molar.

CENTRIC RELATION

Centric relation is a jaw-to-jaw position into which the clinician guides the mandible when the masticatory muscles are relaxed and the condyles are in their uppermost position. In centric relation the opening and closing movement of the mandible for a short distance (B to CR in Figure 1–1) results in rotation around an axis through the condyles. Because a door on hinges rotates only around the hinges, the rotation of the mandible around a transverse axis through the condyles has caused this axis to be called the *terminal hinge axis* of the mandible. This axis is fairly stable. Its location may be pinpointed rather precisely using devices or may be reasonably approximated. The latter results in what is referred to as the *arbitrary hinge axis*.

By relating the mandible and teeth to the patient's hinge axis, the relationship of the mandibular cast can be related to the hinge axis of the articulator. In practice this transfer of information to the articulator is accomplished by guiding the mandible into centric relation and then capturing the relationship between the mandibular and maxillary arches by using heat-softened wax between the occlusal surfaces. Then the wax is cooled and the position of the mandible relative to the maxilla in centric relation is registered in wax. This centric relation registration check bite is then used to relate the mandibular cast to the maxillary cast on the articulator. Thus the mandibular cast is mounted on the articulator in relation to a hinge axis movement of the patient. Thus a terminal hinge axis is common to the patient and the articulator (Fig. 1–7).

With suitable adjustment of the articulator, all the tooth contacts made by a patient in centric occlusion and centric relation, as well as contacts in lateral and protrusive movements, should be capable of being made on the articulator. However, if the casts are mounted in centric occlusion rather than centric relation, retrusive contacts distal to centric occlusion cannot be made. Some articulators are not adjustable and some have no lateral or protrusive movement possibilities. The error resulting from using simple articulators can to a certain extent be compensated for by clinical and laboratory techniques. The articulator to be used should meet the goals for the restorations planned. A simple articulator may be adequate for a small individual restoration but inadequate for multiple restorations.

Centric relation is the position of the mandible in which the condyles are in the uppermost, rearmost position. In this position the condyles have essentially very limited potential for straight lateral movement, and any lateral displacement caused by intercuspation of the teeth may not be acceptable and a functional disturbance may develop. The emphasis on compatibility between centric relation contact and centric occlusion is related to the limited capacity of the temporomandibular joints for lateral and posterior positioning.

In theory, the problem of obtaining centric relation has been solved by every advocate of a particular method. However, experienced operators may obtain centric relation within a small error (~ 0.5 mm) by

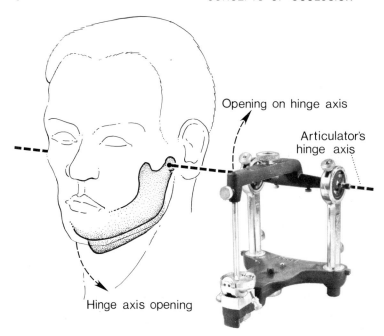

Opening on hinge axis

Articulator's
hinge axis

Figure 1–7. Hinge axis. The terminal hinge axis of the patient and the hinge axis of the articulator represent a frame of reference common to the patient and the articulator.

Hinge axis opening

any method that is compatible with the neuromuscular system. In this respect, an experienced operator knows, or should know, when conditions are optimal. But it is one thing to obtain centric relation and yet another to capture the relationship in order to relate the mandibular cast to the maxillary cast. Although centric relation may not be obtained from a patient for any of the exercises in this manual, a simulated centric relation can be used in all exercises. Such a simulated "centric relation" has limited future clinical value, should be avoided generally in the clinic, and is no substitute for learning to take a centric relation (CR) bite. It is sometimes provisionally used where temporomandibular joint–muscle dysfunction prevents a centric relation registration.

Occlusal Vertical Dimension

Contact vertical dimension as a measure of the height of the lower third of the face has little practical use for individual and multiple restorations. However, occlusal vertical dimension as a component of the occlusal intercuspal position has biologic significance for the maintenance of centric stops and stability of the occlusion. Alterations of the occlusal vertical dimension by bite-raising appliances involving the posterior teeth can result in intrusion of these teeth and extrusion of the anterior teeth, or can cause functional disturbances of the masticatory system such as temporomandibular joint–muscle pain dysfunction, or can cause both these problems. A general principle in restorative dentistry is to maintain contact vertical dimension for single and multiple restorations, or for all complete mouth restorative procedures when it cannot be established that a loss of vertical dimension has occurred.

The occlusal vertical dimension for a set of casts mounted on an articulator is determined by the contact relations of the teeth in the intercuspal position. This vertical relationship should be maintained irrespective of changes made in the occlusal surfaces by the incisal pin and the condylar element supports of the articulator. Rubbing the casts together causes wear of the stone and loss of vertical dimension. It is necessary to make certain that the articulator can be zeroed or set so that the use of its parts (viz., incisal guide table) does not alter vertical dimension. Purposeful alteration of the vertical dimension requires that the mandibular cast be mounted using a centric relation registration and that the incisal pin can be adjusted to meet the center of the incisal table at the increased vertical dimension.

Slide in Centric

According to the freedom in centric concept of occlusal therapy, vertical di-

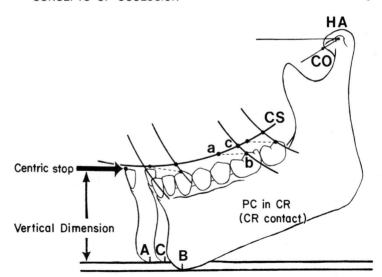

Figure 1–8. Slide in centric. With the mandible in centric relation (*CR*) the movement on the hinge axis (*HA*) results in closure on an occlusal interference at *b*. With the mandible in this position the vertical dimension is *B*. If the premature contact (*PC*) in centric relation is removed, the slide in centric is eliminated and vertical dimension (*C*) is the same as at *A* (centric occlusion). *A* to *C* and *a* to *c* represent freedom in centric or long centric. The vertical dimension at centric relation equals that at centric occlusion.

mension in centric relation must be the same as centric occlusion when all occlusal interferences to closure in centric relation have been removed. In Figure 1–8 vertical dimension is shown in the incisor region in terms of *A*, *B*, and *C*. In Figure 1–9 the position of a point on the teeth (in this instance the first molar) as it relates to the premature contact in CR is given as *b*, the centric relation contact with the premature contact removed as *c*, and the position of centric occlusion as *a*. The factors that influence the amount of the vertical component of a slide in centric (movement from *b* to *a* or *B* to *A* in Figures 1–8 and 1–9) are the height of the premature contact, its anterior-posterior location, and the curve of Spee (*CS*). The discrepancy

between centric relation and centric occlusion would depend upon the position of the condyle in centric relation and centric occlusion in the patient. On the articulator it would be related to the position of the transverse hinge axis (*HA*) or arbitrary hinge axis as transferred to the articulator, and centric occlusion. From a practical standpoint, on the articulator the incisal pin should be in contact with the incisal table at "zero" for both centric relation and centric occlusion. Unless such contact is possible, usually through an occlusal adjustment, it is impossible to use the "long centric pin and table" to develop freedom in centric in individual restorations or anything less than a full mouth reconstruction.

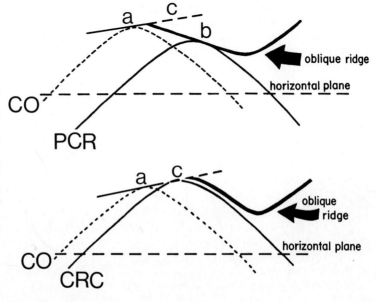

Figure 1–9. Slide in centric. Enlarged view of relationship of *a*, *b* and *c* shown in Figure 1–8. *Upper,* The premature contact (*PCR*) or occlusal interference in centric relation involved the oblique ridge of a maxillary molar. *Lower,* With removal of the PCR interference the slide in centric (*b* to *a*) is removed, leaving freedom in centric or long centric (*c* to *a*).

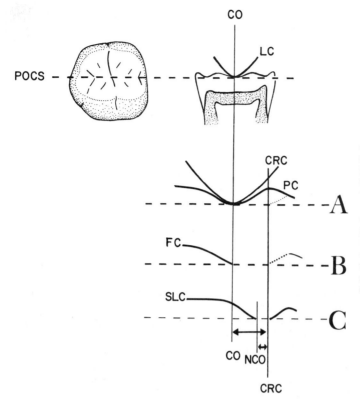

Figure 1-10. Freedom in centric. Lingual supporting cusp (*LC*) occluding on a centric stop in centric occlusion. *POCS* is the plane of occlusion and centric stop in the fossa. Vertical lines for CO and CRC relate to situation at *A, B,* and *C.* With the elimination of the premature contact (*PC*) involving a triangular ridge, freedom of centric (*FC*) from CRC to CO is present as shown in *B.* If the occlusion is restored as in *C* so that a new centric occlusion (*NCO*) is produced, the distance from *CRC* to *NCO* is a shortened long centric (*SLC*), which is 0.5 mm or less.

FREEDOM IN CENTRIC

Freedom in centric is a concept of occlusion in which there is freedom of the mandible to close without interference into contact in centric relation, centric occlusion, and between, and also slightly anterior and lateral to centric relation and centric occlusion. Freedom in centric, or *broad centric* as it is sometimes called, is obtained by an occlusal adjustment or by restorative dentistry that allows the mandible to close into centric without the need for gross neuromuscular responses to occlusal interferences. This centric is developed to place the occlusal forces in the long axis of the teeth.

There are at least two variations on the concept of freedom in centric: (1) centric contact in which the vertical dimension at centric relation is the same as at centric occlusion and there is no alteration of the anterior-posterior relationship of centric occlusion to centric relation and (2) alteration of the distance from centric relation to centric occlusion in a full mouth reconstruction by placing centric occlusion closer (< .5 mm) to centric relation. (The latter is sometimes called *long centric.*) Freedom in centric (Figs. 1–10 and 1–11)

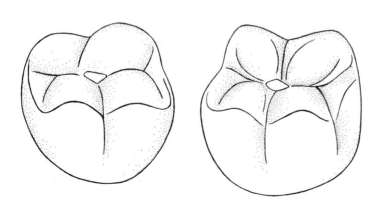

Figure 1-11. Freedom in centric. Relatively flat area in fossa for contact of supporting cusp. Form is related to (1) cuspid guidance and guidance from buccal cusps of posterior teeth (group function) if present, (2) occlusal adjustment, and (3) restorations.

or long centric are not found in the natural dentition. Freedom in centric is produced by an occlusal adjustment and/or single or multiple restorations. Long centric is produced in a full mouth reconstruction in which at least all posterior occlusal surfaces are changed.

GUIDANCE

The control of mandibular movements brought about by the masticatory muscles involves sensory systems that include the periodontium, tongue, temporomandibular joints, muscles, tendons, and skin. In addition, the occlusal surfaces during contact of the teeth not only physically limit closure but also guide the teeth into centric occlusion. As the occlusal surfaces glide on each other, guidance is provided by the morphologic features of the occlusal surfaces. The guidance provided by the cuspid is often referred to as *cuspid guidance,* that provided by the incisors as *incisor guidance,* that provided by the anterior teeth as *anterior guidance,* and that provided by the joints as *condylar guidance.*

Guidance provided by the parts of an articulator varies according to the type of articulator, from simple to so-called fully adjustable types. At this time no articulator can be programmed to duplicate the input from all of the components of the masticatory system. What are called condylar guidance and incisal guidance on an articulator vary greatly in programmability for duplicating guidances on the patient. The path of the condyle is complex, and daily biologic variation makes the task of simulating a path of an articulator very difficult. In effect, the condylar guidance of an articulator does not represent accurately the path of the condyle.

It would be futile to assume that a formula or a set of physical factors could provide a reasonable picture of occlusal guidance. However, the importance of guidance factors is expressed in the many concepts of occlusion that exist. Treatment of the occlusion, then, may be based on the factors that may influence mandibular movement in the most ideal or harmonious way. Something specific may be said about a concept of occlusion by the answer to this question: In jaw movement from centric occlusion, what influences the path of the mandible? The occlusion (teeth and periodontium), the temporomandibular joints, and the neuromuscular system all have varying degrees of influence. Several concepts of occlusion are built around different ideas of the importance of specific influences. Condylar guidance versus tooth guidance is an example.

Another way of indicating subtle differences in ideas as related to concepts of occlusion is to ask the question, In jaw movements from centric occlusion, what influences *should* control the path of the mandible? One concept assumes that all guidance should come from the cuspid (so-called cuspid-protected occlusion). Another concept assumes that all the teeth, at least groups of many teeth, should be in contact in mandibular lateral excursion. This concept of "group function" stresses multiple tooth guidance. The acceptance of such all or nothing concepts of guidance or occlusion is not necessary or desirable. Most important is the health and comfort of the patient.

Sensory inputs from the joints for control of mandibular movement are more significant with the teeth out of contact than the sensory input from the periodontium when the teeth are in contact. However, disharmony between the anatomic and physiologic features of the teeth, joints, and muscles may significantly influence mandibular movements. In the absence of disharmony it appears reasonable that the principal determinants of occlusion for individual or multiple restorations should be the teeth.

ORIENTATION

The *curve of Spee* (also known as *compensating curve* in complete dentures) describes a curve from the tip of the mandibular cuspid to the distobuccal cusps of the mandibular second molar. It does not include the anterior teeth and can be described for each side of the mouth separately.

In Figure 1–12, *FH* refers to the *standard horizontal* or *Frankfort horizontal plane.* It is merely a plane of orientation. However, casts will not be oriented to the Frankfort plane unless both anterior (orbitale) and posterior (porion) bony landmarks are transferred to an articulator. Usually this is not accomplished even with an infraorbital pointer (see Fig. 4–8), which

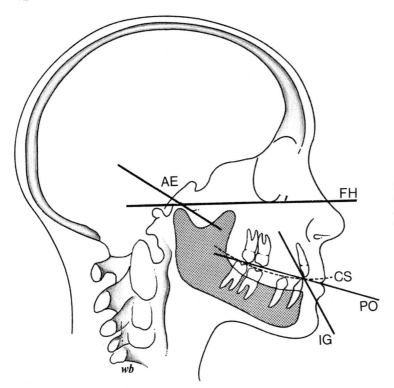

Figure 1–12. Orientation. Plane of occlusion (*PO*); curve of Spee (*CS*); incisal guide (IG); *FH*, Frankfort plane; and *AE*, angle of eminentia.

actually transfers a hinge axis--orbital plane to the articulator. Use of the pointer often results in the maxillary cast being mounted too steeply. Rather, an arbitrary articulator plane is used most frequently.

As shown in Figure 1–13, the vertical or sagittal axis or both of the articulator and patient may be quite different, and the AE shown in Figure 1–12 has little absolute relationship to the condylar inclination

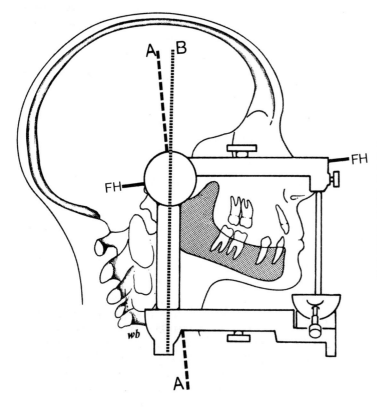

Figure 1–13. Relation of articulator to patient. The plane of occlusion of casts can be related to upper member of the articulator and the plane of occlusion on the patient can be related to the horizontal Frankfort plane (*FH*). In this way the vertical axes of the patient (*A*) and the articulator (*B*) could be related if the orbitale and porion bony landmarks are used and transferred to an articulator (see text).

settings of an articulator. Furthermore, the condyle does not necessarily follow or lie in contact with the bony eminentia. Any angle measured on x-rays may have little meaning to the actual condylar path. There is guidance from the temporomandibular joints and the condyle has a path, but neither are strongly related to the angle of the eminentia, if at all. Recall, when setting the articulator, the meaning of the term condylar guidance of the patient and condylar inclination on the articulator.

BALANCED OCCLUSION

As an articulator is moved with occlusal surfaces making contact, a relationship between five factors has been described by Hanau's Quint or Thielemann's formula. Except for the condylar path, these factors may be developed in complete dentures so that there is harmony between the factors on the articulator and a *balanced occlusion* is established. Balanced occlusion means posterior (bilateral) and anterior tooth contact without interference in all movements. It is developed to prevent tipping of the denture bases in function or parafunction. A balanced occlusion is not necessary or desirable in the natural dentition.

The relationship between the five factors (Thielemann's formula) has been described as follows:

Balanced Occlusion =
   (a constant)
$$\frac{\text{Condylar Guidance} \cdot \text{Incisal Guidance}}{\text{Plane of Occlusion} \cdot \text{Curve of Spee} \cdot \text{Cusp Height}}$$

For example, if condylar guidance (CG) is increased, incisal guidance (G) must be decreased. If the plane of occlusion is increased, the curve of Spee or cusp height must be decreased. Note that these are changes involving the upper or lower compartments (not the numerator or denominator, because this is not a mathematical equation). If the condylar guidance is increased on an articulator (it cannot be done on the human subject), then the plane of occlusion (below the line) must be increased.

The concept of a balance of the five factors of occlusion is applied in relation to complete dentures and to articulation of dentures on an articulator. The usefulness of the five factors is limited in discussing the natural dentition and mandibular movements. For example, when the mandible is moved from centric occlusion forward (a protrusive movement) with the teeth in contact, only the anterior teeth should make contact in the natural dentition. The guidance of the mandible by the cuspids and incisors is not critical in terms of steepness (angulation) for neuromuscular harmony, except for that amount required to prevent contact of posterior teeth in protrusive movement.

The words *must, should, can,* or *may* demonstrate the difference between the requirements of complete denture occlusion and the natural dentition, at least on casts mounted on an articulator. For example, in complete dentures in which the concept of balanced occlusion is applied, cusp height *must* be related to balanced occlusion in considering the plane of occlusion. In protrusive movement, if the plane of occlusion is decreased, the cusp height *must* be increased in order to maintain balanced occlusion. In the natural dentition, however, the concept of no posterior contacts in protrusive indicates that if the plane of occlusion is increased, the cusp height *may* be increased, provided no posterior contact results from the increase.

Considering the importance of the neuromuscular system, joints, and periodontium in mandibular movements, the five factors of occlusion are inadequate to describe all that is involved in the guidance of occlusion. However, the five factors do aid in understanding some of the physical or mechanical relationships of occlusion, especially in the analysis of articulated casts, articulator mechanics, and complete denture fabrication on an articulator.

DETERMINANTS OF OCCLUSION

The factors that determine what the occlusal morphology ought to be in restorations have been called the *determinants of occlusion* (see chart). When referring to complete dentures it has been conventional to refer to condylar guidance, incisal guidance, plane of occlusion, cusp height, and curve of Spee (or compensating curve) as being interrelated for balanced occlusion. However, for the natural dentition such parameters as intercondylar distance, lateral shifting of the condyle, and other condylar factors have been called the con-

Some Determinants of Occlusal Morphology

	Cusp Height	Ridge and Groove Direction		Lingual Concavity of Maxillary Anterior Teeth
		maxilla	mandible	
Intercondylar distance				
greater		→	←	
lesser		←	→	
Working side movement–outward and:				
back		←	→	
forward		→	←	↑
up	↓			↑
down	↑			↓
Condylar inclination–lateral (Bennett)				
greater	↓	←	→	↑
lesser	↑	→	←	↓
Condylar inclination–horizontal				
greater	↑			↓
lesser	↓			↑
Curve of Spee				
greater r	↑			
lesser r	↓			
Anterior maxillary overlap-horizontal				
greater	↓			
lesser	↑			
vertical				
greater	↑			
lesser	↓			
Occlusal plane vs. condylar inclination				
↑ parallelism	↓			
↑ divergence	↑			

← more distal
→ more mesial
↑ increased
↓ decreased

dylar determinants of occlusion — that is, several condylar factors are said to have a significant effect on what the occlusal morphology ought to be in restorations. The concept of condylar-determined occlusion has more relevance to a full mouth reconstruction than to individual restorations. For individual and multiple restorations the occlusion of the other teeth is often more significant than the condyles in determining the occlusion for restorations. However, all components of the masticatory system must be in harmony, including the joints and occlusion.

To meet the goals for tooth determinants of occlusion, restorations may be done totally (amalgam, composites) in cases in which direct carving of the restorative material is done in the mouth. The restora-

tions are formed with the occlusion being related to occlusal contacts during mandibular movements. A technique of making sure that the anatomic occlusal features conform to the patterns of function (or parafunction) on the teeth not being restored is to place softened wax in a cavity preparation and have the patient register in the wax the paths of cusps for various excursions of the mandible. This "wax chew-in" is then used to complete a wax pattern of the restoration using articulated casts.

Also, another way for allowing the existing occlusion to set the anatomic features of a restoration involves the use of articulators in which the articulator condylar elements follow passively the paths set by the occlusion of the casts (Fig. 2–1E). Only a few articulators are designed to fully use this technique because without adequate guidance for the occlusion, which is the case when the patient has no posterior teeth or is completely edentulous, articulators without some means to support the maxillary casts and provide an alternate condylar guidance would be too severely limited to be practical for widespread use. Usually the more adjustable the articulator, the more likely is the possibility for complete articulation of the existing occlusion. Thus the existing occlusion can be used to program the articulator.

Usually, the effect of differing anatomic components (such as intercondylar distance, Bennett movement, and so forth) on cusp height, ridge and groove direction, and degree of concavity of the lingual surfaces of the maxillary anterior teeth are considered in relation to restorative procedures. The effect of differences on restorations must be related to (1) the goals of the concepts of occlusion being applied, (2) averaging versus more precise instrumentation, and (3) whether or not an anatomic component can be changed. The primary objective is the development of an occlusion that is compatible with the neuromuscular system.

Unit 1 Exercises

Directions: Fill in or circle the correct answer as appropriate.

1. Centric occlusion is not considered to be a stable position because _____

   _____

   _____

2. Centric occlusion involves a three-dimensional position of the centric stops

   and thus dictates _____

   _____

   _____ .

3. Centric relation is an unstrained position that occurs around the terminal

   _____ . It is a frame of reference used to _____

   on an articulator. A stable jaw position in centric relation is enhanced when

   there are no premature contacts in _____ .

4. Rest position is defined as a _____ position related to

   _____ dimension, and to _____ space.

   Contact vertical dimension is dependent upon _____

   _____ .

5. In making dentures using an articulator, five physical factors of occlusion are

   related in the concept of _____ occlusion.

6. The Frankfort horizontal plane passes through the _____

   and the _____ . The angle of eminentia, measured from the

   Frankfort plane on a cephalogram, (is/is not) the condylar guidance angle on

   an articulator.

7. The angle of the eminentia does not accurately describe the path of the

   _____ in protrusive or lateral movements.

8. Thielemann's formula dealing with various factors of occlusion is more re-

   lated to _____ factors than to neuromuscular factors, more

   related to _____ occlusion than to _____

   occlusion, and more useful on an _____ than in the _____

   _____ dentition.

9. The term "normal occlusion" refers to an _____ of _____

_____, not universally found, not the "norm," not necessarily related to an absence of occlusal interferences and not necessarily "ideal," but often used as an orthodontic goal.

10. All mandibular movements occur within an _____ of movements.

11. In normal occlusion the mesial lingual cusp of the maxillary first molar occludes where?

_____

12. The path that the distal buccal cusp of the right mandibular first molar projects from centric occlusion on the maxillary first molar in right working movement is toward the (mesial, distal, buccal) palate.

Unit 1 Test

1. Rest position changes with head position:

   a. but contact vertical dimension is responsive to changes in rest position
   b. and should be used to relate the mandibular cast to the maxillary cast because it is a functional position
   c. a and b
   d. and should be considered even in a single restoration
   e. a, b, and d

2. Freedom in centric:

   a. has anterior-posterior and lateral dimensions
   b. occurs in almost everyone
   c. would improve the dental health of most adults
   d. is best when about 0.5 mm long
   e. all of the above

3. Centric occlusion:

   a. can be used to relate the maxilla to the mandible without error
   b. can be used to mount casts that will have no occlusal interferences in centric occlusion, but will have in centric relation
   c. is not always anterior to centric relation
   d. is not found in animals
   e. all of the above

4. When casts are to be mounted in centric occlusion, the use of wax for the registration will:

   a. not prevent error due to compressive forces
   b. not influence the neuromuscular system
   c. prevent occlusal interferences in centric occlusion
   d. not usually produce anterior-posterior error in the mounting
   e. all of the above

5. Centric occlusion:

    a. is maximum intercuspation of the teeth
    b. is the initial contact position of the open-and-close clench
    c. is best determined with stone casts
    d. is almost always correct if casts are mounted in centric relation
    e. all of the above

6. Centric occlusion:

    a. may be influenced by the force of clench or bite
    b. may not be registered on mounted casts correctly because of hard wax used for the interocclusal registration
    c. may not be obtained correctly on casts because of incorrect use of impression material
    d. may be influenced by the temporomandibular joints
    e. all of the above

7. Freedom in centric can be:

    a. found rarely, if ever, in the natural dentition
    b. developed in an occlusal adjustment
    c. formed in restorations
    d. developed in complete dentures
    e. all of the above

8. A tooth with increased mobility (jiggling tooth):

    a. may be adapting to an occlusal interference
    b. could be a response to an initial interference elsewhere in the mouth
    c. a and b
    d. will show progressive injury and thus traumatic occlusion
    e. a, b, and d

9. A full crown restoration is seated with cement. The "filling" feels "high" and requires grinding. The reason for the interference could be:

    a. thickness of the film of cement
    b. case mounted in centric occlusion
    c. poor temporary restoration and some extrusion of the tooth
    d. impressions taken after clenching or mouth open for one-half hour for crown preparation
    e. all of the above

10. Occlusal interferences may interfere with:

    a. swallowing and speaking
    b. chewing
    c. a and b
    d. centric occlusion function
    e. a, b, and d

11. Concerning mastication of food:

    a. Tooth contacts rarely occur in centric occlusion
    b. Tooth contacts occur frequently and regularly in centric relation
    c. An ideal occlusion is a requisite for masticatory efficiency
    d. It is done primarily in a border position
    e. None of the above

12. The greater the outward-upward direction of the rotating condyle in the vertical plane, the greater the Bennett movement, and the greater the intercondylar distance:

    a. the greater the lingual concavity of the maxillary anterior teeth
    b. the shorter the cusps
    c. a and b
    d. the more distal the ridge and groove direction on the maxillary teeth
    e. a, b, and d

13. The lesser the Bennett movement:

    a. the longer the cusps
    b. the more distal the ridge and groove direction
    c. a and b
    d. the greater the maxillary anterior lingual concavity
    e. a, b, and d

14. Which of the following factor(s) will affect: (1) cusp height, (2) ridge and groove direction, and (3) lingual concavity of the maxillary anterior teeth (all three):

    a. direction of rotating condyle (horizontal plane)
    b. Bennett movement
    c. intercondylar distance
    d. direction of rotating condyle (vertical plane)
    e. all of the above

15. An "ideal" occlusion:

    a. refers to an arrangement of teeth and esthetic and functional goals
    b. requires that the arrangement of teeth be conducive to occlusal stability
    c. a and b
    d. is the same as a normal occlusion (angle Class I)
    e. a, b, and d

Unit 2

Adjustable Articulators: Parts and Functions

An articulator is a mechanical device for joining casts of a patient's dental arches so that diagnostic and restorative procedures can be carried out away from the patient. The range of articulators varies from simple hinge-like devices to sophisticated, highly adjustable instruments. Unfortunately, none can faithfully duplicate the complex movements of the mandible. In any case, the type of articulator to be used should be consistent with the goals of occlusal therapy.

The instrument used here is the Hanau H2–PR, a semi-adjustable articulator based on the average dimensions of ~110 millimeters. It is assumed that the articulator is suitable in dimensions for the average patient. The PR adjustment, or protrusive-retrusive adjustment, facilitates the mounting of casts in centric relation.

INTRODUCTION: UNIT OBJECTIVES AND READINGS

The objectives of this unit are to identify the components of functions of a semi-adjustable articulator. Several behavioral objectives are included.

A. Objectives
1. Be able to identify all the parts and function of the parts of the articulator.
2. Be able to discuss the limitations of articulators.
3. Be able to discuss the use of the incisal guidance.
4. Be able to describe the use of the long centric incisal pin and table.
5. Be able to discuss the differences between arcon and nonarcon types of articulators.

B. Readings (optional)

Beck, H. O.: A clinical evaluation of the arcon concept of articulation. J. Prosthet. Dent. 9:409, 1959.

Weinberg, L. A.: An evaluation of basic articulators and their concepts: Part I, Basic concepts. J. Prosthet. Dent. 13:622, 1963.

Weinberg, L. A.: An evaluation of basic articulators and their concepts: Part II, Arbitrary, positional, semiadjustable articulators. J. Prosthet. Dent. 13:645, 1963.

TYPES OF ARTICULATORS

There are numerous adjustable articulators designed to meet one or more requirements (Fig. 2–1). Articulators are classified in several ways, but a practical and simple classification system is: (1) simple or straight line, (2) average value, (3) semiadjustable, and (4) "fully" adjustable. Classifications 3 and 4 are combined into the category of adjustable articulators, since no articulator is actually fully adjustable. Another classification divides adjustable articulators into arcon and nonarcon type articulators. The term *arcon* comes from an articulator designed by Bergstrom called an ARCON (ARticulator CONdyle).

The adjustable articulators in common use in this country are: (1) Hanau H2, (2) Whip-Mix, (3) Denar, and (4) TMJ. Articulators commonly found in Europe are the Dentatus (very similar to Hanau H2) and the Gerber Condylator. In the arcon type instrument the condylar elements are on the vertical axis and condylar guidances are on the upper (maxillary) member. The Hanau H2, Dentatus, and Condylator are nonarcon types sometimes referred to as *axle-type articulators.*

All articulators in common use have an upper and lower member, with the upper

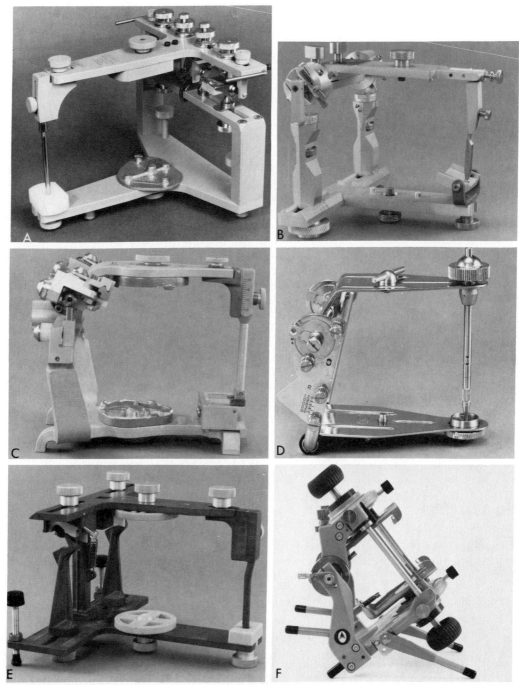

Figure 2–1. Adjustable articulators. "Fully" adjustable articulators: *A,* Stuart, *B,* Simulator, *C,* Denar. Semi-adjustable articulators: *D,* Gerber, *E,* TMJ, *F,* Gnathomat.

member holding the maxillary cast. Since the upper member is movable, the movement of the maxillary cast is the reverse on the patient in whom the mandible moves. This relationship is sometimes confusing to the student at first, but the reversal becomes less and less of a problem in a short period of time.

All the adjustable articulators in common use utilize a position on the terminal hinge as a mounting position for the lower casts (centric relation [CR] check bite) and will accept a face bow transfer to orient the maxillary cast to condylar elements of the articulator.

The articulator and face bow are used to join a patient's casts in such a way that mandibular movement and occlusal contacts can be simulated. The simulation of mandibular movements and occlusal relations has two problems: (1) use of a stable, reproducible frame of reference, and (2) use of a device (articulator) that will adequately simulate jaw movements.

HINGE AXIS

The frame of reference common to articulator and patient is the terminal hinge axis, which is determined (1) by palpation, (2) *mechanically* with a device called a kinematic face bow, and (3) *arbitrarily* by manual or automatic measurement 12 to 13 mm anterior to the tragus. The errors involved in these determinations are dis-

cussed in Unit 8 and elsewhere.* How the hinge axis is determined will be covered in Unit 7.

The *registration* of the axis means locating the hinge axis points on each side of the face. These two points must be related to the maxillary arch and then the maxillary cast related to the hinge axis points on the articulator. This transfer is made with a *face bow*, a device that *transfers* the relationship between the hinge axis of the patient and the maxillary arch to the articulator through the mounting of the maxillary cast to the articulator. (See "Quick Look at Face Bow Function," Unit 4.)

THE HANAU H2–PR ARTICULATOR

On the Hanau H2–PR the upper member has two condylar elements (Fig. 2–2). Through the elements and the upper member is a shaft (or axle) corresponding to the transverse hinge axis. The condylar elements glide in slots called the *condylar guidance* (Fig. 2–3). The guidance, called the horizontal condylar guidance, may be inclined to simulate the path of the condyle (forward and downward). As indicated in Unit 1, the condylar guidance inclination in degrees is not the angle of the eminentia nor the path of the condyle in

---

*Bosman, A. E.: Hinge Axis Determination of the Mandible. Leiden, Stafleu and Tholen B. V., 1974.

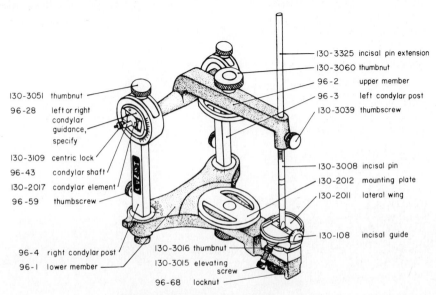

Figure 2–2. Hanau H2 articulator–parts.

degrees. The inclination in degrees is a relative measure, not an absolute value related directly to another angle, i.e., angle of eminentia.

The upper member of the articulator may be locked in a forward position against a mechanical stop (called a centric stop) in "centric." If the mandibular cast is mounted in centric relation and the upper member locked (with the centric locks) against the centric stops, the upper member is locked in centric relation. If the mandibular cast is mounted in centric occlusion, the upper member will be locked in centric occlusion.

When the upper member is locked in "centric" (centric relation or centric occlusion), that is, when the condylar elements are locked against the centric stops, movement of the condylar guidance through various inclinations will produce no changes in the upper member. When the spacer and centric stops are in position on the Hanau H2–PR and the condylar elements are against the centric stops, the condylar shaft of the upper member is centered in the condylar guidance (Fig. 2–3).

Inasmuch as the Hanau H2–PR articulator does not accept a kinematic face bow or hinge axis locator, it is impossible to transfer the true hinge axis of the patient to the hinge axis of the articulator. The hinge axis of the Hanau H2–PR articulator is the center of the condylar shaft when the condylar elements are against the centric stops (Fig. 2–3). As will be seen later, the practical use of an arbitrary hinge axis leads only to small errors that are acceptable for most treatment procedures.

If the mandibular cast is mounted in centric relation (and a slide in centric exists in the patient), when the casts are moved into centric occlusion (centric locks, 153–104 loosened), the condylar shaft will not be centered in the condylar guidance slot.

The Hanau H2–PR has a provision for Bennett movement — that is, for possible side shift movement of the mandible. It is an averaging type of movement and does not attempt to produce an immediate side shift. Bennett movement is called lateral condylar inclination on the Hanau H2–PR and is determined from the horizontal condylar inclination (Fig. 2–4A) by a formula provided on the underside of the base of the articulator (Fig. 2–4B).

The formula for the lateral condylar guidance on the Hanau H2–PR has never been tested for its validity. Whether or not there is such a relationship between horizontal condylar guidance inclination and Bennett movement (lateral condylar guidance) is a moot question. However, the Bennett movement appears somewhat limited on the H2–PR (30°) in contrast to the Dentatus (40°).

Of particular importance in the use of the Hanau H2–PR is the correct manipulation of the upper member to obtain the Bennett movement. In right lateral excursion (Fig. 2–5), the condylar shaft (axle housing) moves laterally, while the condylar element remains in contact with the working side centric stop. At the same time the edge of the condylar shaft housing on the balancing side remains in contact with the condylar element. The balancing side element moves away from the condylar stop (Fig. 2–6) in lateral movements.

In a "fully" adjustable articulator, a side shift is programmed in a specific way with

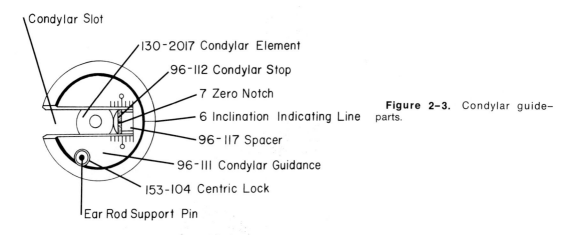

Condylar Slot

130-2017 Condylar Element

96-112 Condylar Stop

7 Zero Notch

6 Inclination Indicating Line

96-117 Spacer

96-111 Condylar Guidance

153-104 Centric Lock

Ear Rod Support Pin

Figure 2–3. Condylar guide-parts.

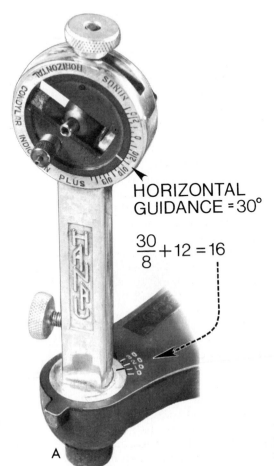

HORIZONTAL
GUIDANCE = 30°

$$\frac{30}{8} + 12 = 16$$

A

Figure 2–4. Setting lateral condylar inclination. *A*, correlation between horizontal inclination setting and lateral inclination; *B*, formula on underside of articulator for setting lateral inclination.

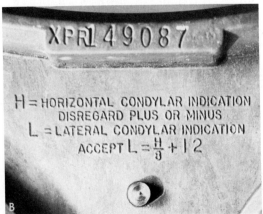

XPR 1 49087

H = HORIZONTAL CONDYLAR INDICATION
DISREGARD PLUS OR MINUS
L = LATERAL CONDYLAR INDICATION
ACCEPT $L = \frac{H}{8} + 12$

B

IN RIGHT LATERAL EXCURSION

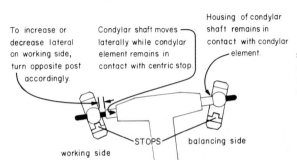

To increase or decrease lateral on working side, turn opposite post accordingly.

Condylar shaft moves laterally while condylar element remains in contact with centric stop.

Housing of condylar shaft remains in contact with condylar element.

STOPS

working side   balancing side

Figure 2–5. Lateral shift action. Proper lateral shift of upper member of the Hanau H2 articulator requires the condylar shaft housing to remain in contact with the condylar element on the balancing side during lateral movements.

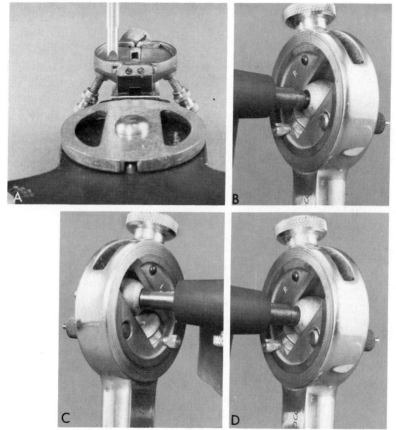

Figure 2–6. Position of the components of the H2 articulator to obtain Bennett movement. *A*, incisal pin in a position of right working movement; *B*, correct position of condylar shaft housing and condylar element on the right side in a right working position; *C*, correct contact between housing and element on the left side in a right working position; *D*, incorrect contact relationship between shaft housing and condylar element on the right side for right working movements.

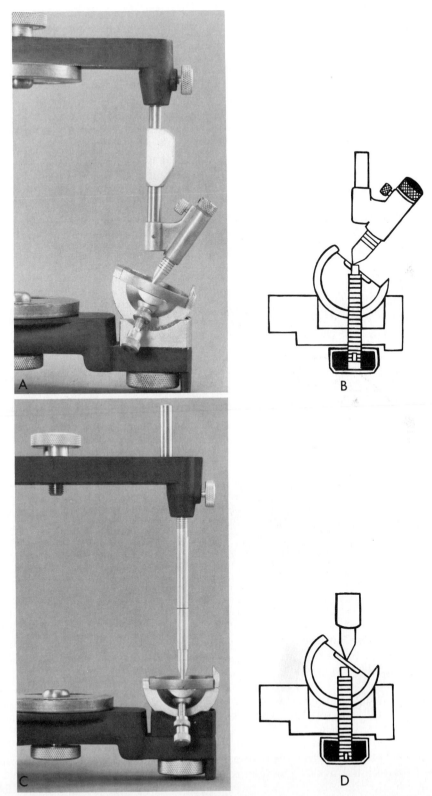

Figure 2-7. Incisal pin and guide table. *A*, Schuyler long centric pin; *B*, schematic of Schuyler pin and table; *C*, straight pin; *D*, freedom in centric (FC) pin out of function.

the teeth out of contact so that no guidance is obtained from the teeth. In contrast, one articulator (TMJ) uses guidance obtained from the patient's teeth to fabricate the condylar fossa out of soft acrylic on the articulator.

The incisal guide table on the Hanau instrument is used to simulate guidance by the anterior teeth. The incisal guidance can be adjusted for a positive inclination of 60° and a negative inclination of 20°. The articulator may have a guidance table with a "long centric" table (Fig. 2–7A, B) and an adjustable incisal pin (Fig. 2–7A, B). At this time the straight pin can be used (Fig. 2–7C) and the long centric table pin placed below the surface of the table (Fig. 2–7D). The incisal table inclination and the inclination of the lateral wings are set to replace the tooth guidance in order to prevent wear of the stone casts and to provide guidance when tooth structure or teeth are not present to provide the guidance.

ADJUSTMENT OF THE ARTICULATOR

Before the articulator (Hanau H2–PR) is adjusted, all working parts must be clean and oiled and freely movable. Wax, plaster, dried oil, and dirt will prevent the condylar element from moving freely in the condylar guidance slots. Observe the condylar element for freedom of movement, checking to see that the centric lock (Fig. 2–8D) does not impede movement into lateral and protrusive positions. The condylar guidance should be free to move from 0° to 70° to 0° again.

Protrusive-Retrusive Components

The Hanau H2–PR articulator has a protrusive-retrusive adjustment feature that will allow the maxillary cast to be moved forward and backward for various reasons. The primary uses are to simulate a centric relation position and to allow the casts to be locked in centric occlusion when the mandibular cast has been mounted in centric relation.

Prior to use, the protrusive-retrusive feature must be adjusted to a "zero" centric. A spacer (96–117) is placed in front of the centric stop (96–112) as shown in Figure 2–8A. When the spacer is inserted, the condylar element cannot go into a retrusive position, only into centric or protrusive position. This spacer must be removed for retrusive adjustment. The spacer is not removed at any time in procedures in this manual.

The PR is at "zero" centric when the spacer is inserted and the centric stop (96–112) is turned clockwise until the back of the centric stop is against the spacer, and the notch (7, shown in Fig. 2–8A) on the serrated edge of the centric stop is lined up with the zero line (6, Fig. 2–8A) on the condylar guidance inclination (Fig. 2–8B). The centric stop is locked into position by the lock screw on the inner front surface of the condylar guidance (Fig. 2–8C).

When the condylar element is against the centric stop and the underedge of the serrated edge of the centric stop is aligned with the zero of the PR calibration, the condylar shaft is centered in the condylar guidance. Because the condylar element is centered, no movement of the upper member will take place when the condylar guidance inclination is changed. With the condylar elements in any position but "zero," that is, any protrusive or retrusive position, there will be movement of the maxillary cast when the condylar guidance is moved.

Each spacer and centric stop has been individually fitted to the condylar guidance slots. Do not lose the spacers and do not attempt to interchange the stops and spacers. When not in use on the articulator, the spacers should be kept in the articulator case, taped to the lid.

Each full turn of the centric stop is 1 millimeter and each line on the serrated edge indicates one-quarter millimeter. The calibration on the condylar guidance for the protrusive-retrusive adjustment is set in millimeters.

Articulator Alignment

Before mounting casts on the Hanau H2–PR articulator, it is necessary to adjust the articulator to a correct starting point. There are adjustable components of the articulator that during normal use may accidentally loosen or may be altered purposefully according to the needs of the restorations being fabricated. It is then necessary to return these adjustable components to their correct starting points be-

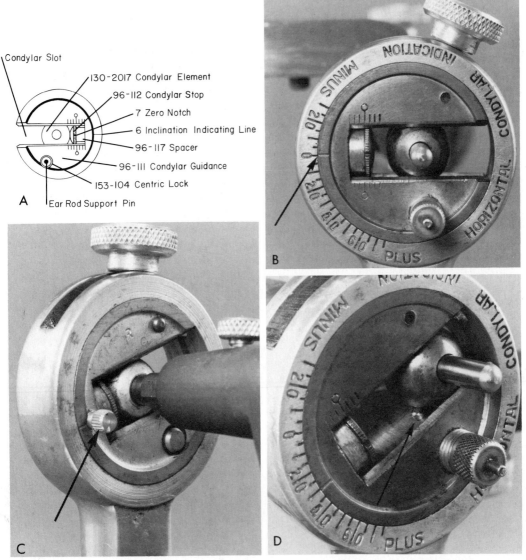

Figure 2–8. Parts of Hanau H2–PR condylar guide. *A*, identification of parts; *B*, condylar inclination set at zero; *C*, condylar stop lock nut; and *D*, pin in condylar slot. This is activated by the condylar element centric lock.

fore mounting casts for a new and different procedure.

The articulator must be checked for anteroposterior ("zero" centric) and lateral malalignments. Because the level of the incisal pin affects the anterior positioning of the upper member of the articulator, it should be adjusted so that the top of the pin is flush with the upper surface of the upper member of the articulator, and the blade of the incisal pin should be positioned perpendicular to the long axis of the articulator. Adjustments of the incisal pin are made by loosening the incisal pin thumbscrew. Setting the incisal guide table and lateral wings at 0° will also

facilitate determining the articulator malalignment. This adjustment is made by releasing the corresponding lock nuts.

If the PR adjustment is not fixed in "zero" centric, the thumbscrew on the inner surface of the condylar guidance should be released and the necessary rotations of the centric stop should be made until "zero" centric is indicated. If the PR adjustment is not at "zero" centric on both sides of the articulator, the incisal pin will not be centered laterally. This type of malalignment should be differentiated from that caused by a bent incisal pin, bent axle (condylar shaft), or incorrect centering of the condylar shaft housings.

QUICK LOOK AT PROCEDURE FOR CHECKING
ZERO ON THE HANAU H2–PR ARTICULATOR

1. Set horizontal condylar inclination at "0" (Fig. 2–9A). Loosen the thumbnut (C) and move the condylar guide so that the indicating line (A) is set at zero.

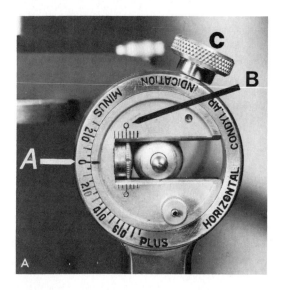

2. Set condylar stop at "0" (Fig. 2–9A, B). Loosen the lock screw and set the condylar stop so that the flat edge of the centric stop is in line with "0" of the PR calibration (B). Set the notch (N) on the rim of the condylar stop to "0" (Fig. 2–9B).

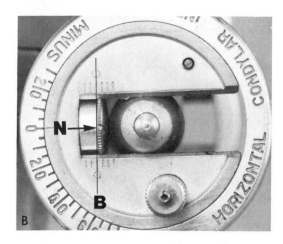

3. Set lateral condylar inclination at "0" (Fig. 2–9C). Loosen thumbnuts and rotate the condylar posts until the bench marks on the post and articular base are at "0."

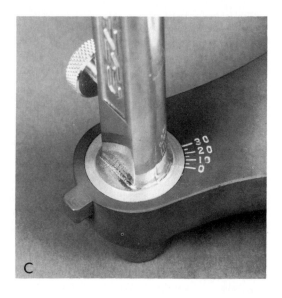

4. Set the incisal table inclination at "0" (Fig. 2–9D, E). Set the incisal table to "0" (Fig. 2–9D) and turn the elevating screw counterclockwise to reduce the lateral wings to "0" (Fig. 2–9E).
5. Check that the incisal pin is centered (Fig. 2–9D, E, F). With the top of the incisal pin flush with the upper member of the articulator, the blade of the incisal pin should be centered laterally (Fig. 2–9E) and anterior/posteriorly (Fig. 2–9D) on the incisal table. Check with articulating paper (Fig. 2–9F).

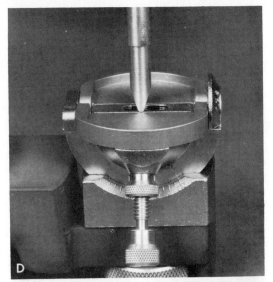

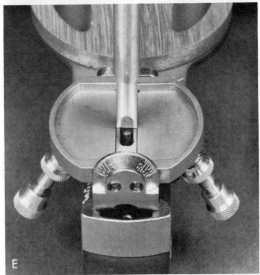

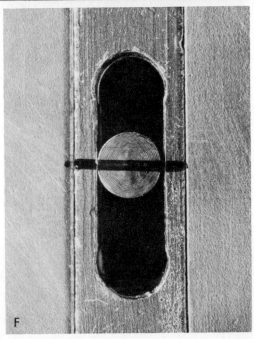

Figure continued on following page

6. Check that the upper member is centered (Fig. 2–9G). If there is lateral movement of the upper member when locked in centric and/or the incisal pin is not centered laterally, the condylar shaft housing must be adjusted.

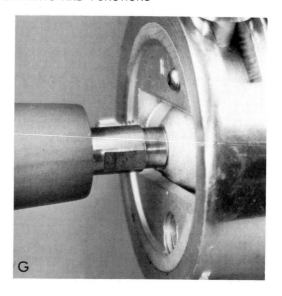

G

Zeroing the Hanau H2–PR Articulator

To zero the H2–PR articulator, nine adjustments must be checked to read zero degrees, the incisal pin must be centered anteroposteriorly and laterally, and all the thumbnuts must be locked.

Unlock the thumbnut on the condylar guidance. Rotate the condylar guidance back and forth from 0–70 degrees to see if it moves freely. Set the scribed line on zero and lock the thumbnut.

Unlock the centric lock. Also unlock the centric stop using the thumbscrew found on the inner surface of the condylar guidance. Unless it is already positioned, correctly rotate the centric stop until its flat undersurface (mesial aspect) is aligned with the zero reading on the protrusive-retrusive (PR) scale. In this position the undersurface should be in contact with the spacer in the condylar slot and the deep zero notch on the centric stop should be aligned with the zero on the horizontal inclination scale. After the alignment, pull the upper member of the articulator forward and tighten the centric locks bilaterally. The condylar elements must rest against their centric stops before the centric locks are tightened.

Unlock the thumbscrew on the condylar post. Rotate the post back and forth. Do they move freely? Set the scribed line at zero and tighten the thumbnut.

Unlock the lock nut at the base of the incisal table. Rotate the table to see if it moves freely. Set its scribed line at zero and tighten the lock nut.

Reduce the elevating screw of the lateral wings until they are at their zero setting. Lock the thumbnut found on the elevating screw. Check the length of the incisal pin: it should be 108 mm in length.

Check the anteroposterior centering of the incisal pin as follows: Loosen the thumbnut found on the front of the upper member. Slide the pin so that its top is flush with the upper member. Position the pin so that the thumbscrew is tightened against the flat surface found on the upper part of the pin. Tap the pin (attached to upper member) against the incisal table. Check the anteroposterior centering of the pin with articulating paper (Fig. 2–9E). If the blue mark does not appear in the anteroposterior center of the table it may be due to manufacturing error or the pin may be long or bent, the table too high, or the centric stops not set at zero. In any case you will have to raise or lower the pin until it does contact the anteroposterior center of the table. The distance between the upper and lower members of the articulator should be 108 to 110 mm when measured behind the incisal table with the pin correctly positioned. The height of the incisal table above the lower member should be about 12 mm.

The pin must also be centered laterally. If it is not centered laterally and the incisal pin is the correct length and not bent, the condylar shaft housing will have to be adjusted. Loosen the two locking thumb-

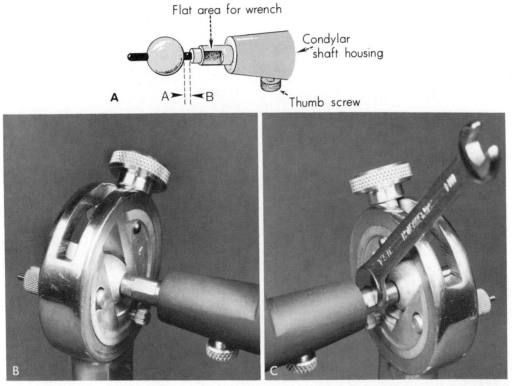

Figure 2–10. Zeroing the H2–PR articulator. *A*, schematic of components of condylar element, shaft, and lock for housing. The surface of the housing (*B*) should just make contact with condylar element (*A*) when the condylar elements are in contact with the centric stops; *B*, housing in contact in centric; *C*, use of wrench to change position of housing when thumbnut has been loosened.

nuts for the condylar shafts (axles) found on the undersurface of the upper member (Fig. 2–10*A*). Check the "play" (side-to-side movement) of the upper member and the lateral movements of the pin on the table. The play should be less than 0.1 mm but greater than zero, and the incisal pin blade should make contact between the inner edges of the lateral wings of the incisal guidance (Fig. 2–10*B*). To correct for excessive play or for incorrect lateral placement, the condylar shafts can be adjusted by rotation with a 7/32 inch wrench (Fig. 2–10*C*). With correct adjustment the pin will be centered laterally on the table and the condylar shaft housing will barely touch the condylar element. Tighten the two thumbscrews and check the lateral centering of the pin and the play in the upper member.

Considering some of the problems of vertical dimension* with articulated casts

*A change in the dimension between upper and lower members of the articulator and loss of some or all centric contacts between mounted casts.

if the articulator is not properly zeroed, the following are the most common:

1. If the incisal pin is not centered anteroposteriorly a change in the vertical dimension will occur if the incisal table is moved from a zero setting (Fig. 2–11).

2. If the incisal pin is laterally centered but not anteroposteriorly centered, that is, if it is distally placed and a positive inclination of the incisal table is required, the edge of the pin may make contact with the edge of the table before an adequate protrusive movement can be accomplished.

3. If the pin has not been centered laterally when the lateral wings are elevated, a change in the vertical dimension will occur.

4. If the condylar shafts and condylar elements are not at the centers of the condylar guides for all inclinations as shown in Figure 2–11*B*, a change in the vertical dimension will occur at differing inclinations of the condylar guidance. (This is a manufacturing error if centric stops cannot be set correctly at zero.)

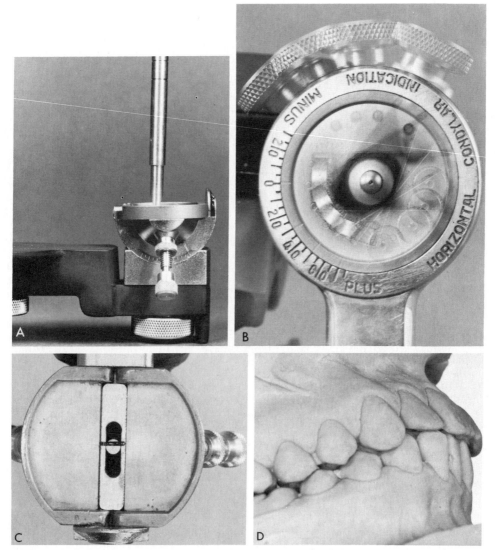

Figure 2–11. Incorrect articulator zero and effect on vertical dimension. *A, C,* anterior posterior setting of incisal pin incorrect; *B,* hole at end of axle remains stationary if condylar element is positioned correctly. However, if the pin is set incorrectly as in *A, C* or the condylar element not set at zero as in *B,* the upper member of the articulator will be raised as in *D,* and cause disclusion of the teeth (increased vertical dimension).

ARCON AND CONDYLAR ARTICULATORS

There are many arcon and nonarcon types of articulators for articulating casts, but three of the most commonly used articulators are the Hanau H2–PR, the Whip-Mix, and the Denar. The Denar, shown in Figure 2–12*A, B,* is an arcon type semi-adjustable articulator, whereas the Hanau H2 is a condylar type semi-adjustable articulator (Fig. 2–12*C, D*). Another Hanau articulator, the Hanau *158–4,* is an arcon instrument (Fig. 2–12*E, F*). On the arcon articulator the condylar guides are attached to the upper member and the condylar elements to the vertical axis of the lower member.

A major difference between the two types of articulators relates to the removal of the upper member. On the arcon type, the upper member of the articulator rests on the condylar elements, whereas on the condylar type (H2–PR) the upper member is locked in the condylar guide slot. In this

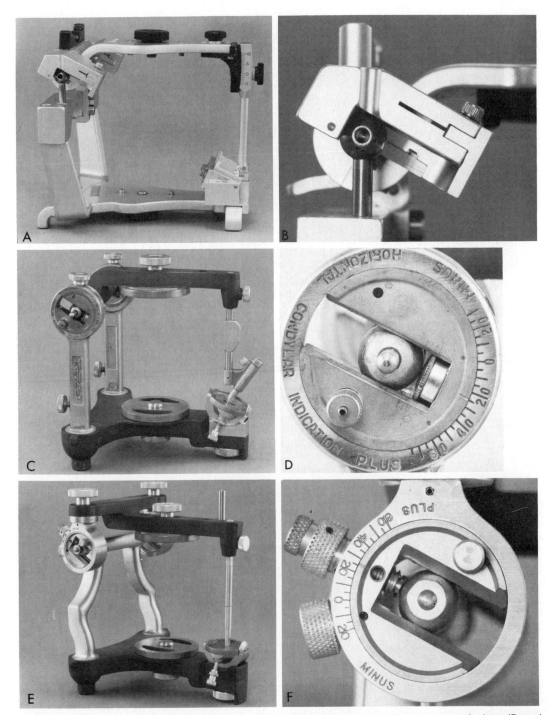

Figure 2–12. Arcon compared with condylar articulators. *A*, semi-adjustable arcon type articulator (Denar); *B*, upper member rests on condylar element; *C*, Hanau H2–PR condylar articulator; *D*, condylar element fixed to upper member; *E*, Hanau arcon type articulator; *F*, upper member rests on condylar element within condylar slot.

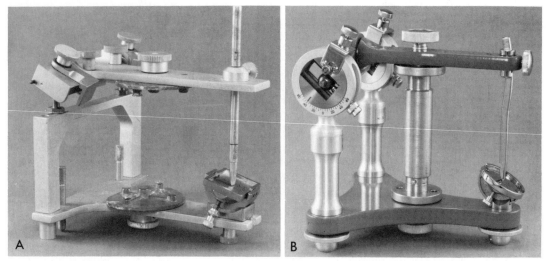

Figure 2–13. Arcon compared with condylar articulators. *A*, Whip-mix semi-adjustable articulator; *B*, Dentatus semi-adjustable articulator.

respect when using an arcon type instrument the operator must be careful that the guiding surface of the upper member is always in contact with the condylar element.

Some arcon instruments, such as the Whip-Mix (Fig. 2–13A), have provisions for changing the intercondylar distance. On the Whip-Mix the adjustment is some-what analogous to small, medium, and large.

The condylar guidance on the condylar type of instrument, the Hanau H2–PR, is set with a protrusive interocclusal record because it will not accept a lateral check bite.

As already indicated, the lateral inclination on the H2–PR is set with the formula

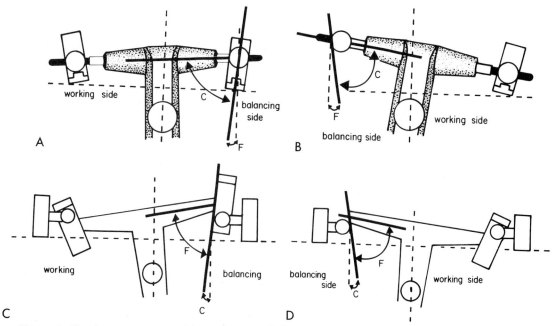

Figure 2–14. Arcon versus condylar articulator. *A, B,* condylar articulator. *C, D,* arcon articulator (see text).

on the underside of the base of the articulator. However, with the Dentatus (Fig. 2–13B), another condylar type instrument, the lateral condylar inclination can be set with lateral check bites. On the Dentatus, the lateral inclination setting can be set as high as 40°. On the arcon type instrument (Whip-Mix) the horizontal condylar inclination and Bennett angle can be set from interocclusal wax records made with the mandible in both right and left lateral protrusive movements.

As shown in Figures 2–14 and 2–15, differences do exist between arcon and condylar articulators. Differences in angles are evident, such as differences in the angle between the condylar guidance and the shaft housing or hinge axis of the upper member. The angles are reversed; i.e., in one instrument an angle is fixed, whereas in the other instrument the angle changes. In these figures, F refers to fixed angle; that is, the angle between the axis and the condylar guide does not change in a given movement. C refers to a changing angle, and CP to changing occlusal plane. The instruments produce the same motions on the basis of condylar guidance, being the result of interaction between a condylar ball and an inclined plane. Remember that in an arcon articulator, the condylar *guide* moves with the upper member; in a nonarcon articulator, the condylar *ball* moves with the upper member.

In Figures 2–15A and 2–15B the difference between an arcon and condylar articulator in the sagittal plane is shown. As the condylar instrument is opened (vertical dimension increased), the occlusal plane (CP) changes but the condylar guidance angle remains fixed. On the arcon type instrument the condylar guidance angle changes as the articulator (upper member) is opened.

In restorative procedures that involve "raising the bite" or "opening the bite" (increasing contact vertical dimension), most condylar type instruments (semiadjustable) are not usually recommended because of apparent limitations in full mouth reconstruction. No advantage has been shown to be present in using arcon instruments for complete dentures, although there may be some advantage with fully adjustable articulators when changes in vertical dimension are to be undertaken. (Most so-called fully adjustable articulators [instruments with three-dimensional movement potential] are usually arcon instruments.)

According to some writers, the arcon type reflects physiologic conditions more fully than does the condylar type. However, clinical superiority for the arcon instrument has not been demonstrated. Many clinicians do not accept any practical differences between the arcon and condylar types of articulators, whether they are semi- or fully adjustable.

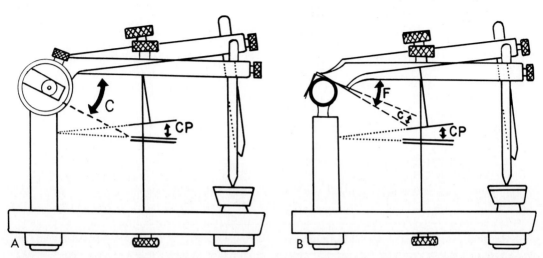

Figure 2–15. Arcon compared with condylar articulator. A, condylar type; B, arcon type of articulator (see text).

Unit 2 Exercises

1. If the incisal pin is not centered anteroposteriorly, what problem may arise in setting the incisal table?

2. If the pin is not centered laterally, what problem may arise in setting the lateral wings of the incisal guide table?

3. If lateral play in the upper member is present, what effect could it have on dental restorations fabricated on the articulator?

4. Which articulator adjustments affect anteroposterior positioning of the incisal pin?

5. Which articulator adjustments affect lateral positioning of the incisal pin?

6. When waxing a molar restoration on an arcon type of articulator such as a Whip-Mix articulator, what effect would be produced by not having the condylar element in contact with its guiding surface?

7. Why might an articulator with a varying intercondylar distance be considered hypothetically to be more accurate than an articulator with an average
intercondylar distance?

_____

_____

_____

8. Identify the components in Figure 2–16:

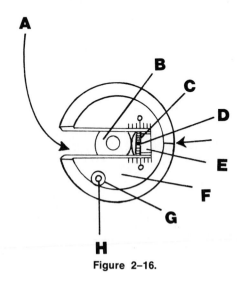

Figure 2–16.

9. Name two errors that may alter the vertical dimension of mounted casts.

_____

_____

10. Name two possibilities that can alter the lateral positioning of the incisal
pin.

_____

_____

11. Give three possible explanations for the anteroposterior position of the
incisal pin being altered.

_____

_____

12. Which manufacturing error may result in a change of vertical dimension
when a change in the condylar inclination is necessary for mounting of the
mandibular cast?

_____

_____

Unit 2 Test

1. The Hanau articulator (H2–PR):

   a. should be zeroed with the incisal table set at zero
   b. should be centered with the lateral inclinations set at zero
   c. a and b
   d. should be centered with the condylar element centric stop set at zero on both sides
   e. a, b, and d

2. If casts are mounted in centric occlusion with the articulator at zero and then the spacer removed and the centric stop moved anteriorly (forward) on the H2–PR articulator, the:

   a. incisal pin will not be centered on the table (anteroposteriorly)
   b. change will provide simulated centric relation position for the condylar elements, but condylar guidance will not produce the same result
   c. the most relative retrusive position of the mandibular cast would be 3 mm
   d. centric occlusion remains the same
   e. all of the above

3. When an articulator (H2–PR) is adjusted correctly, all of the following are correct except:

   a. the housing for the condylar shaft rests tightly against the surface of the condylar element
   b. the condylar element seats in direct contact with the centric stop with the incisal pin centered
   c. the maxillary cast will usually have adequate room to move in a protrusive direction
   d. the condylar elements should not bind on the shaft (axle) housing
   e. the lateral condylar guidance may be set from 0° to 30°

4. Which of the following may affect lateral positioning of the incisal pin:

   a. centric stop adjustment
   b. lateral guidance
   c. condylar guidance setting
   d. type of contact of condylar element and shaft (axle) housing
   e. all of the above

5. The Whip-Mix and Hanau H2–PR are similar in that:

   a. an ear rod face bow is used to mount the maxillary cast
   b. some type of interocclusal record (wax bite) is used to set condylar guidance
   c. a and b
   d. both have provisions for adjustment of intercondylar distance
   e. a, b, and d

6. Relative to arcon versus condylar articulation:

   a. on the Hanau H2–PR the angulation in protrusive movement of the condylar slot is constant to the lower member
   b. during protrusive movement, the angulation changes between the upper member and the condylar slot of the Hanau articulator
   c. a and b
   d. on an arcon articulator (Whip-Mix), in protrusive, the lower member remains constant in relation to the condylar slot
   e. a, b, and d

7. The differences in clinical results that can be obtained using the Hanau H2–PR and the Whip-Mix articulators:

   a. are not clinically significant for most dental procedures
   b. are most significant for extremes of intercondylar distance
   c. a and b
   d. are not significant for fabrication of most dentures
   e. a, b, and d

8. The articulator shown in Figure 2–17 is:

   a. a condylar type
   b. an arcon instrument
   c. fully adjustable
   d. a and c
   e. b and c

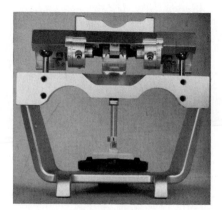

Figure 2–17.

9. In Figure 2–18 the maxillary cast is moving into:

   a. right working, incorrectly
   b. right working, correctly
   c. left working, incorrectly
   d. left working, correctly
   e. impossible to indicate, not sufficient information

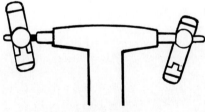

Figure 2–18.

10. The movement of the condylar inclination 0 to 70° (Fig. 2–19A, B) would result in:

    a. a movement upward of the maxillary cast
    b. a movement downward of the maxillary cast
    c. upward and forward movement of the maxillary cast
    d. downward and forward movement of the maxillary cast
    e. none of the above

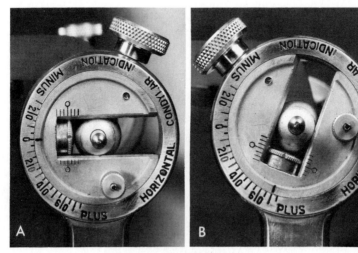

Figure 2–19.

Unit 3

Semi-adjustable Articulators: Anterior Guide

As previously indicated, the incisal guide (incisal table and incisal pin) of an articulator is a physical simulation (sometimes referred to as mechanical equivalent) of the physical guidance provided by the anterior teeth. Although the name implies only guidance set by the incisor teeth, the incisal guide also may include canine guidance when provisions have been made for it in the incisal table. Perhaps a better term to use is anterior guide (table) rather than incisal guide (table), especially where lateral protrusive guidance is possible. Because the mounting of casts will not be discussed until Unit 7 and occlusal adjustment until the completion of Unit 11, the practical aspects of Part 2 of this unit should be delayed until then.

Part 1

INTRODUCTION: UNIT OBJECTIVES AND READINGS

The objectives of this unit are to introduce the theory of the incisal guide, its use, and its limitations. Behavioral objectives are included.

A. Objectives
   1. Be able to identify parts of the incisal guide.
   2. Be able to describe the function of the incisal table and pin for general use (Part 1) and how to use the Schuyler pin and table to develop freedom in centric (Part 2).
   3. Be able to demonstrate the limitations of the incisal guide of the articulator.
   4. Be able to prepare a customized anterior (incisal guide) table.

B. Reading (optional)
   Schuyler, C. H.: An evaluation of incisal guidance and its influence in restorative dentistry. J. Prosthet. Dent. 9:374, 1959.

ANTERIOR GUIDANCE: BIOLOGICAL CONSIDERATIONS

It would be incorrect to attempt to isolate the influences of the anterior parts of the masticatory system on mandibular movement as if no other influences exist. It is also incorrect to suggest that the physical guidance of the teeth is the most important controlling factor in anterior guidance when anterior guidance is the sum of a number of sensory as well as physical contact inputs to the control of occlusal relations of the anterior teeth. However, it is true that the contact relations in protrusive and lateral protrusive excursions are those aspects of guidance easiest to visualize.

It is not unusual for functional disturbances to develop in the masticatory system as a result of what may appear to be minor physical or esthetic changes or both in the anterior teeth. Entrapment of the mandibular incisors by encroachment on centric occlusion in new maxillary anterior restorations is a frequent cause of functional disturbances. In effect, the patient cannot swallow or chew in centric occlusion, and distal displacement of the mandible results in temporomandibular joint–occlusal disharmony, especially in the presence of a premature contact in centric relation.

There is no evidence that the anterior teeth protect the posterior teeth or that occlusal contacts on anterior teeth should be heavier than on posterior teeth. The control of forces on all teeth, separately and in groups, depends on a number of factors, many of which are at this time hypothetical.

Steepness of incisal or cuspid guidance is not important for neuromuscular harmony. Actual steepness should harmonize with the existing occlusion. An arbitrary increase to avoid group function of posterior teeth is not indicated. An arbitrary increase of incisal guidance to ensure posterior disclusion in the absence of functional disturbances in itself may lead to occlusal dysfunction in certain instances such as anterior open bite.

ANTERIOR GUIDE TABLE AND PIN

The functions of the anterior guidance system of an articulator are (1) to serve as a guide for the establishment of the occlusal morphologic features of restorations for anterior teeth relative to protrusive and lateral protrusive movements in a comprehensive oral rehabilitation, (2) to prevent wearing down of the teeth with loss of vertical dimension when casts are articulated, (3) to prevent distortion of waxed restorations and loss of vertical dimension during the waxing stage of restorative procedures, and (4) to aid in setting cuspid guidance during waxing of an occlusal bite plane splint. A number of tables and pins have been developed to take into account one or more of these functions.

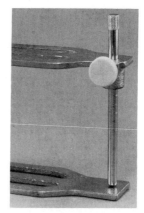

Figure 3–1. Anterior guide table and pin. Incisal pin without incisal guide table.

Some act only to maintain vertical dimension in centric (Fig. 3–1); some consist of flat planes fixed at an angle to each other for a fixed angle of lateral guidance but having a provision that allows change in the angle of protrusive guidance. In others comprehensive adjustments can be made on tables that have adjustable flat planes for lateral guidance as well as have the capacity to be adjusted for steepness of incisal guidance in protrusive movements of the mandible (Fig. 3–2). In one, a shallow saucer-shaped thin metal sheet can be flexed for a combination of curvatures for lateral and protrusive guidances (Fig. 3–3);

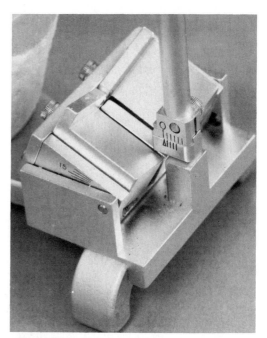

Figure 3–2. Adjustable incisal guide and pin. Incisal table adjustment limited to flat planes and angles.

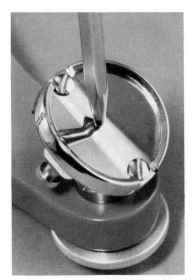

Figure 3–3. Adjustable incisal guide. Guidance set by thin metal sheet so that all directional changes are smooth.

others are holders for quick-setting acrylic, which is ploughed into the guidance set by contact relations of the teeth (Fig. 3–4).

The rationale for the various designs is directed toward providing a guidance that is consistent with economics and use of the guide table and pin. For example, the contact between two cuspids or two incisors in lateral or protrusive movements is not represented usually by a flat plane — the facial surface and cusp tip of the mandibular cuspid or incisor are curves, and during movement points or areas on these surfaces follow the curvatures of the lingual surfaces of the maxillary cuspids or incisors. Whenever a standard or "fully"

adjustable table and pin do not allow adequate contact between contacting teeth that are to be used to set the pattern of anterior guidance, it is possible to provide curves for guidance of the pin rather than flat planes by using a customized guide made of quick-cure acrylic. Thus flat planes of an adjustable table allow only limited contact between guiding inclines of teeth, whereas curved planes that are custom formed by following the guiding inclines of the teeth may provide a more specialized guidance when required. In effect, a "fully" adjustable table and pin may not be as completely adjustable as one that is customized. When there is a broad freedom in centric present or significant curvature to tooth guidance, a customized anterior guide is required.

Incisal Pins

As shown in Figure 3–5, incisal or anterior guidance pins differ principally according to whether or not provisions for changing vertical dimension are included. If contact vertical dimension is to be changed, it is necessary to adjust the pin so that the tip is centered again after the change has been made.

Several methods have been devised to provide the capacity for change in vertical dimension: the curved pin on the Dentatus (Fig. 3–5A), the curved pin holder on the Denar (Fig. 3–5B) and TMJ articulators (Fig. 3–5C), and the off-set type pin on the Hanau (Fig. 2–7A) and Simulator articulators (Fig. 3–5D). The mechanics of these pins will be discussed in relation to the Schuyler pin and table.

Providing Anterior Guidance

Providing anterior guidance with an incisal pin and table varies with the requirements of the restorative problem. The procedure of establishing an anterior guidance in a case in which no remaining anterior guidance is present not only involves attending to esthetics but also making certain of harmony between the anterior and posterior occlusion. This procedure is far more difficult than setting the incisal guidance in cases in which most of the guidance from anterior teeth still remains. Setting the incisal guidance to protect the teeth, to maintain vertical

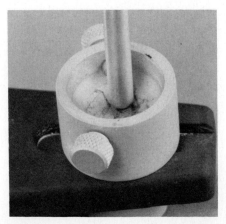

Figure 3–4. Adjustable incisal guide. Cup used to hold quick cure acrylic to form a custom incisal guide.

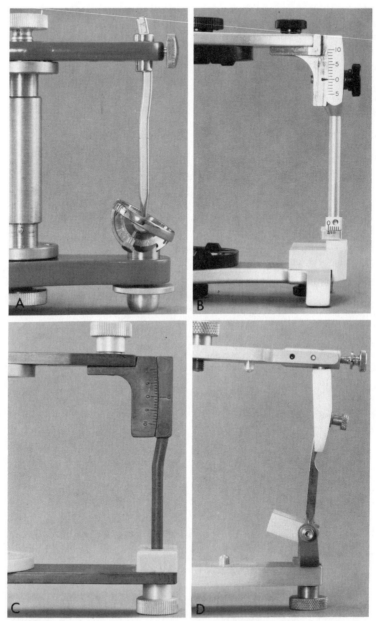

Figure 3–5. Adjustable incisal guide pin. Incisal pins that are adjustable to compensate for changes in vertical dimension: *A*, Dentatus; *B*, Denar; *C*, TMJ; *D*, Simulator.

dimension, and to wax anterior restorations for individual and multiple restorations is by far the most common use of the incisal pin and table. Several methods for carrying out these functions are available and will be discussed in Part 2.

SETTING AN ADJUSTABLE ANTERIOR GUIDE

Because casts have not been mounted in the articulator, the present discussion is principally for orientation. However, this section will be referred to in Unit 7.

Setting the Incisal Table

An adjustable table such as the Hanau table and straight pin (Fig. 3–6A) is set according to the following steps:

1. Open the centric locks, the incisal guide thumbscrew, and the elevating screw for the lateral incisal guide.

2. Push the upper member of the artic-

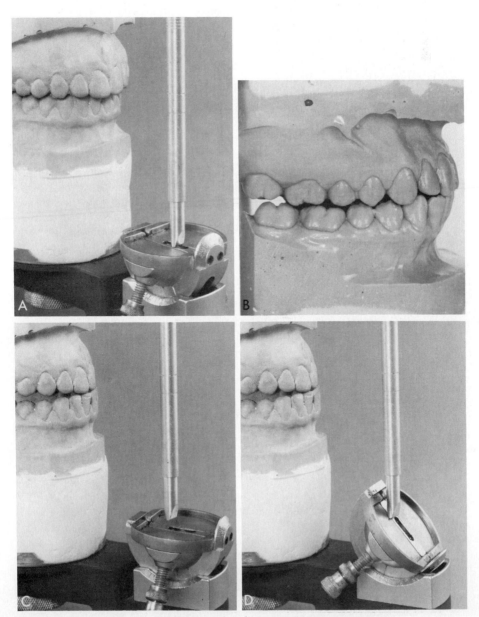

Figure 3–6. Setting anterior guide table. *A*, Center pin on table; *B*, move maxillary cast into protrusive relation; *C*, pin should not be in contact with table; *D*, elevate table to make contact with pin.

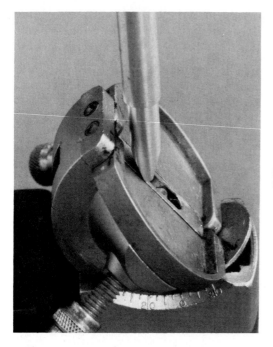

Figure 3–7. Protrusive position of pin. Pin should be free of contact from rim of table in protrusive movement.

ulator backward until the incisal edges of the teeth are in an end-to-end relationship (Fig. 3–6*B*). The pin will not be in contact with the incisal guide table (Fig. 3–6*C*).

3. Raise the incisal table until it touches the incisal pin (Fig. 3–6*D*).

4. Tighten the incisal guide thumbscrew. If the incisal guidance of the stone casts is too steep for the articulator to accept, the table must be customized. The incisal pin should not hit the edge of the table and lose contact in protrusive (Fig.

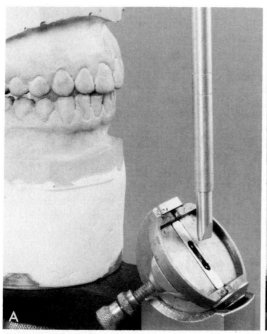
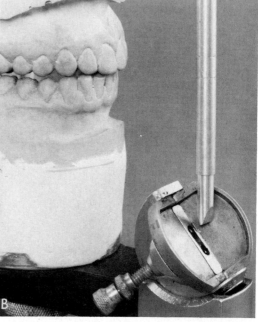

Figure 3–8. Setting lateral wings. *A*, Place casts in cuspid-to-cuspid contact; *B*, raise lateral wing to just make contact with pin. Repeat for right side.

3–7). If this happens, the incisal guidance must be customized.

5. Move the articulator laterally until the cuspids are in an end-to-end position (Fig. 3–8A) and raise the lateral wing of the incisal table with the elevating screw until the wing makes contact with the incisal pin (Fig. 3–8B). Lock in position with the lock nut on the elevating screw. Repeat for the opposite side.

Part 2

Part 2 of Unit 3 is concerned with concepts of adjustable incisal pins that can be adjusted to different vertical dimensions yet can make contact at the center of the table. A second objective is to introduce the customizing of the incisal guide table. Another objective is to discuss the use of the Schuyler long centric table and adjustable pin. This part of Unit 3 should be covered after the casts have been mounted and an occlusal adjustment done.

CUSTOMIZED GUIDES

Customized Incisal Cup

With a cup type of guidance (Fig. 3–9), the pin is raised a few millimeters off the bottom of the cup so that there is no contact with the metal and there is sufficient thickness of acrylic to prevent tearing during movement of the pin.

Fill the cup with a dough-like mixture of quick-cure acrylic. Then guide the upper member of the articulator through all lateral and protrusive movements so that the patterns of movements are traced in the soft acrylic. Once the acrylic is set it can be trimmed with a bur and the guidance can be used.

Customizing an Adjustable Table

A Schuyler incisal pin and table may be customized by elevating the freedom in centric (FC) or long centric pin for several millimeters (Fig. 3–10A) and elevating the table and wings slightly to prevent dislodgement of the acrylic. A dough-like mixture of TMJ* or Hanau† acrylic (or other type of quick-cure acrylic that can be used to form a customized incisal table) is applied to the table, with care taken that some of the material provides a "lock" to hold the acrylic in position. With the teeth in contact, guide the upper member of the articulator through all movements necessary to form the guidance in the acrylic (Fig. 3–10B).

Customizing the Schuyler table with elevation of the FC pin is a rapid method for taking into account freedom in centric for single or multiple restorations, especially when a significant lateral slide has been eliminated. Thus when an occlusal adjustment has been done so that freedom in centric exists, the customized incisal guidance will reflect the occlusal area. However, if a full mouth reconstruction is being done and no tooth contacts of freedom in centric are present to act as a guide for customizing an incisal table, the dimension of the anteroposterior and lateral freedom in centric is determined by setting the Schuyler pin and table, i.e., without customizing.

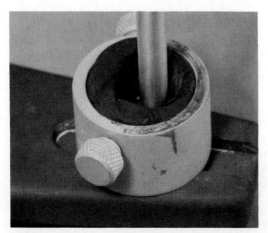

Figure 3–9. Customizing incisal table (see text).

*"tmj" Fossa and Tray Acrylic, TMJ Instrument Co., Inc.

†Hanau Pantacrylic, Teledyne Dental, Hanau Division.

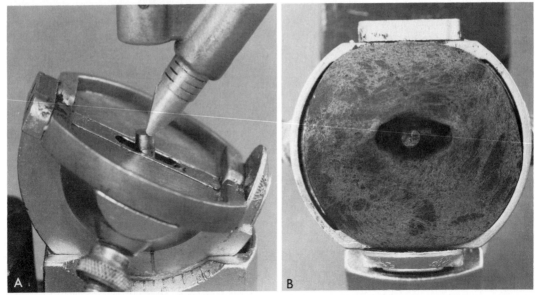

Figure 3–10.   Customizing Schuyler table (see text).

USE OF SCHUYLER PIN AND TABLE

An objective of this section is to introduce the function of incisal guidance and the use of the Schuyler pin and table

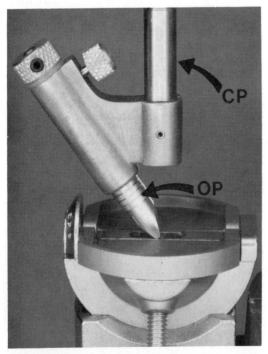

Figure 3–11.   Schuyler adjustable guide pin. *CP,* center pin (incisal guide pin); *OP,* off-set pin to adjust for change in vertical dimension.

as it relates to freedom in centric. The Schuyler pin and table (Fig. 3–11) are used in the development of long centric or freedom in centric. Other articulators have methods for accomplishing the same thing.

Pin

Another closely related objective is to introduce the use of an adjustable pin to compensate for a change in vertical dimension, but only the use of the Schuyler pin will be discussed at this time.

Vertical Dimension

Considerable emphasis has been placed on "zeroing" the articulator, including the anteroposterior and lateral position of the incisal pin on the incisal table. One of the reasons for anteroposterior centering was to provide room for protrusive movements without the pin making contact with the back edge of the incisal table, especially with angulation of the table close to maximum (60°).

Another reason for emphasis on zeroing the pin relates to its path on the incisal table when it is not centered (anteroposteriorly) and when the incisal table and lateral wings are not at zero. A change in the anteroposterior position of the pin will

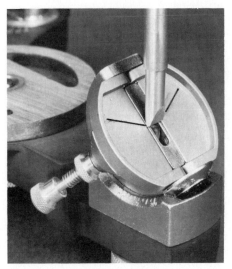

Figure 3–12. Influence of table on path of incisal pin. Elevating the incisal pin guide table results in a change in the angle of the path.

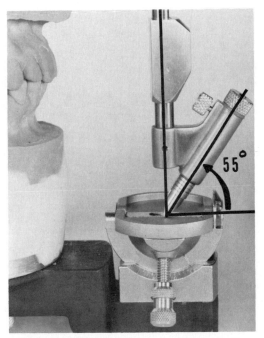

Figure 3–14. Angle of Schuyler off-set pin. These angles provide for effective adjustment for changes in vertical dimension.

result in a different gothic arch tracing (Fig. 3–12) from that found at anteroposterior zero, (Fig. 3–13). If there is an increase in vertical dimension (extending the central pin from the upper member and increasing the length of the off-set pin) to be undertaken in a reconstruction, with a CR check bite, and with an occlusal splint, the pin must be adjusted to zero

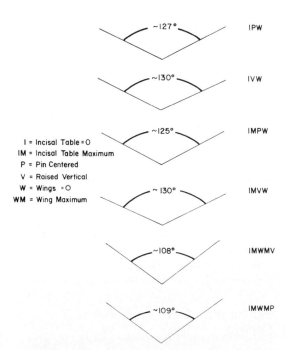

I = Incisal Table = 0
IM = Incisal Table Maximum
P = Pin Centered
V = Raised Vertical
W = Wings = 0
WM = Wing Maximum

~127°   IPW

~130°   IVW

~125°   IMPW

~130°   IMVW

~108°   IMWMV

~109°   IMWMP

Figure 3–13. Influence of the anterior guide adjustment on the path of the incisal pin.

(anteroposterior) when the increase in vertical is being made.

Compensation for changes in vertical dimension may be accomplished with the Schuyler pin by changing the off-set incisal pin (OP) along with the vertical central pin (CP), as shown in Figure 3–11. At anteroposterior zero the off-set pin makes an angle of 55° with the horizontal and 35° with the central pin (Fig. 3–14). The angle of 35° is fixed, but the angle that the off-set pin makes with the horizontal can change from 55° at anteroposterior zero to a larger number, depending upon how much the vertical dimension is increased.

The way in which the central pin and the off-set incisal pin compensate for a change in vertical dimension is shown in Figure 3–15. A line drawn through the anteroposterior center of the incisal table at 55° to the horizontal (IT = incisal table = 0) is essentially coincident with the arc of a circle with radius (r) having its center at the hinge axis (HA) of the articulator. The vertical dimension is changed by lifting the upper member of the articulator (UMA). When moved from contact with the incisal table, the upper member moves from a to b to c. There is very little error involved from a to b, and it is only when approaching c in vertical dimension that

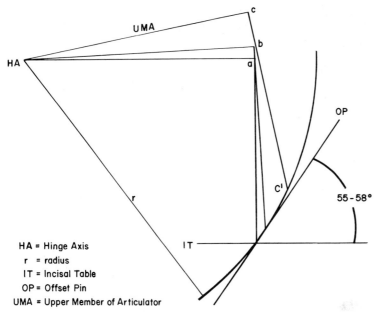

Figure 3–15. Function of offset pin. *OP,* off-set pin tangent to arc of curvature at different vertical dimensions at *a* and *b* (see text).

HA = Hinge Axis
r = radius
IT = Incisal Table
OP = Offset Pin
UMA = Upper Member of Articulator

point c^1 departs greatly from line OP (off-set pin). At point c^1 the angle has increased from 55° to 58°. When the off-set pin is set at the broad zero (0) line (Fig. 3–16) and the pin anteroposteriorly centered, the distance between the upper and lower members of the articulator should be very close to 110 mm. When the central pin is dropped to increase the vertical 2 to 3 mm,

the off-set pin must be adjusted (counterclockwise) to extend the pin to the third or fourth mark beyond the zero mark on the off-set pin (Fig. 3–16). The length of the off-set pin and the anteroposterior width of the table set the mechanical limits of compensating for an increase in vertical dimension.

Another method of compensating for changes in vertical dimension is to use a curved surface for the front of the incisal pin (Fig. 3–17*A,B,C*). The curve formed by letters a, b, and c would be approximated by letters a, b, and c in Figure 3–15.

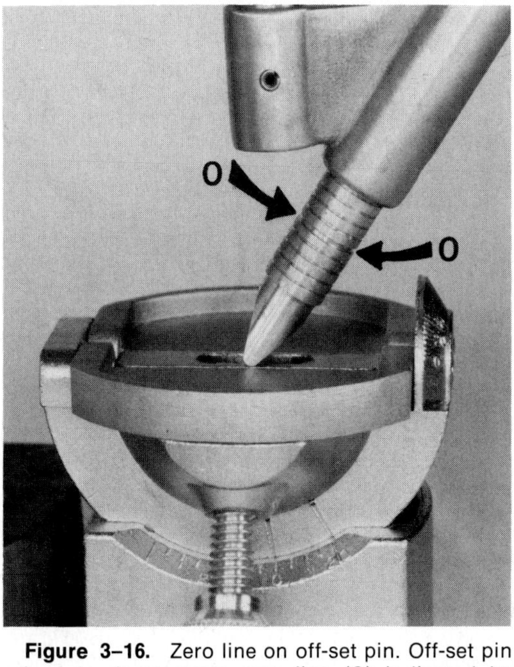

Incisal Guide Table

The Schuyler table is made with an adjustable (FC) pin (Fig. 3–18) to provide for freedom in centric or long centric. When this pin is below the surface of the table it has no influence. When raised, it can be used to establish both an anteroposterior and lateral freedom of up to about 2 mm, depending on pin elevation (Fig. 3–18*C*). The degree of elevation of the lateral wings influences the degree of lateral freedom: the higher the lateral wings of the incisal table, the less the lateral freedom.

Setting the FC Pin for Freedom in Centric

The setting of the FC or long centric pin will depend upon the magnitude of the

Figure 3–16. Zero line on off-set pin. Off-set pin raised to demonstrate zero line (O) indicated by arrows.

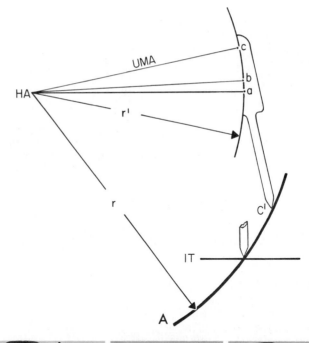

Figure 3–17. Function of curved pin. Curvature acts to keep pin related to a constant radius for a short distance (see text).

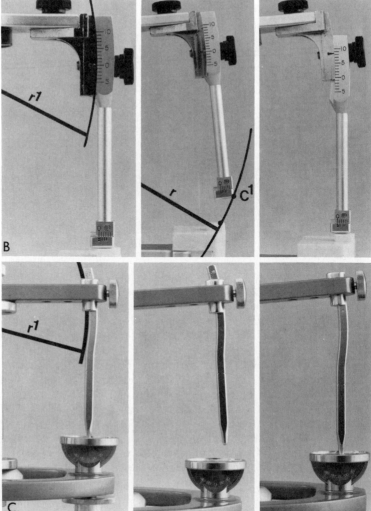

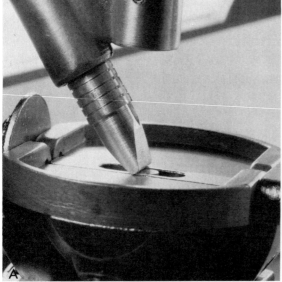
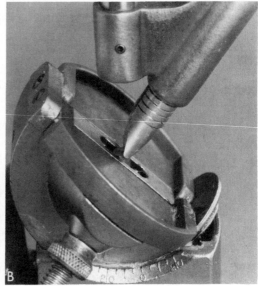
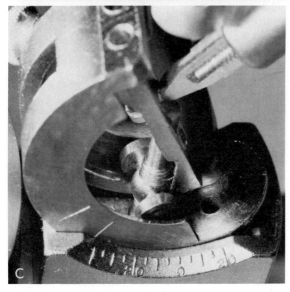

Figure 3–18. Schuyler pin and table. *A*, off-set pin in contact with table and FC pin; *B*, off-set pin raised into position; *C*, gibel of off-set pin must be in position to function properly.

freedom obtained with an occlusal adjustment. Thus the amount of discrepancy between centric occlusion and centric relation determines the magnitude of the freedom in centric that can be obtained by an occlusal adjustment. This amount of freedom will be reflected in individual or multiple restorations that are being waxed. However, in a full mouth reconstruction the magnitude is determined by the setting of the FC pin. Thus the clinician, not the occlusal adjustment, determines the amount of freedom in a full reconstruction. The lateral component of freedom in centric for individual and multiple restorations is dictated to a large extent by the occlusal anatomy of the adjustment and by the elevation of the lateral wings of the incisal guide table.

An idea of the procedure for setting the FC pin is shown in Figure 3–19, in which a numerical sequence is followed. Loosen the thumbnut, locking the incisal guide table. Raise the incisal guide table (IT) to 60° as indicated by 2 (Fig. 3–19*B*). Note that the off-set pin encroaches on the face of the table at *a* and causes the incisal pin to be raised as in Figure 3–19*C*. Because of the encroachment at *a* the pin is raised as shown at 3. Also, there is an increased vertical dimension as seen between the central incisors at 3 (Fig. 3–19*D*). The raised table (ITR) is set at a maximum of 60°. The central incisal pin (6) and the

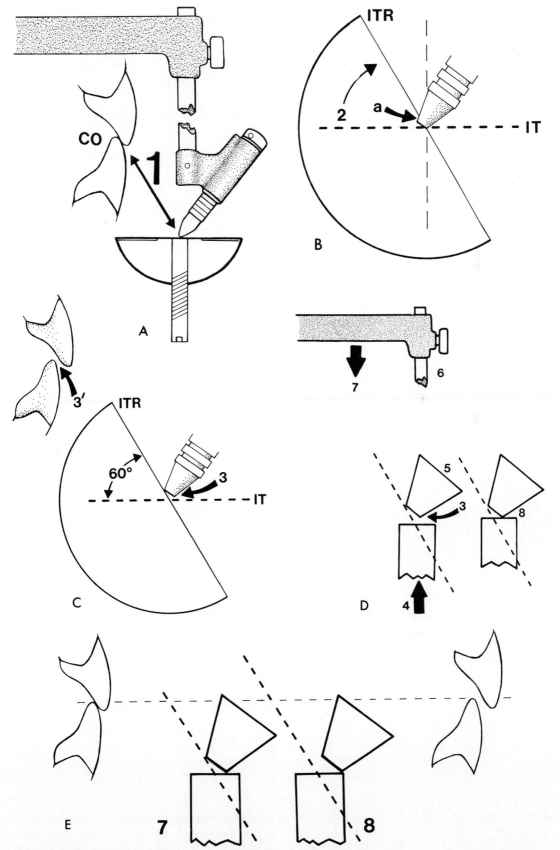

Figure 3–19. Setting Schuyler pin and table for long centric or freedom in centric function (see text).

off-set pin (5) are unlocked and the maxillary cast occluded into centric occlusion by pressure on the upper member of the articulator (7). The FC pin is raised to contact with the off-set pin (4). Adjust both 6 and 5 as required to contact the off-set pin and the face of the incisal guide table (8) and provide freedom in centric. Unlock the condylar locks and rotate the condylar stop clockwise to zero. Remove the maxillary mounting and note the position of the off-set pin in centric occlusion (7) and in centric relation (8). The ability to move without hindrance from 7 to 8 is the anteroposterior freedom in centric (Fig. 3–19E).

Exercise: Simulated Setting of FC Pin

Set the PR adjustment clockwise 1 mm or insert 1 mm shims between the condylar elements and condylar stops (Fig. 3–20). Lock the condylar locks. In the laboratory situation it is possible to use casts mounted in a simulated centric relation (Unit 7) provided that an occlusal adjustment is done (Unit 9). However, in the clinical situation the occlusal adjustment for freedom in centric is done first, then an impression taken, and the casts mounted in centric relation.

Zero the vertical pin and off-set pin with articulating paper (Fig. 3–21). Elevate the FC pin above the table about 1½ mm (Fig. 3–21C) and elevate the incisal table as required for incisal guidance.

The FC pin should be elevated sufficiently to provide 1½ to 2 mm of space on the pin forward of the inclined face of the incisal table (Fig. 3–22A). If the FC pin is too high for the angle of elevation of the incisal table, the adjustment by the off-set pin will result in rough contact between the off-set pin and table (Fig. 3–22B).

There should be no space between the off-set pin and table (Fig. 3–22C). Hold onto the articulator as shown in Figure 3–23A, and with the thumb and forefinger move the incisal pin up and down (casts in centric occlusion), and adjust the off-set pin for the desired anteroposterior position on the FC pin (Fig. 3–23B). With the casts in centric occlusion, adjust the central incisal pin and off-set pin until the face of the off-set pin makes contact with the face of the incisal table (Fig. 3–23C). Check to see that centric stops have been

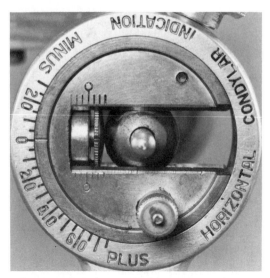

Figure 3–20. PR adjustment for simulated mounting in centric relation with casts in centric occlusion.

maintained in centric occlusion. Remove the casts from the articulator.

Reset the condylar stop clockwise to zero (or remove the shims) and move the condylar elements into the simulated centric relation position (Fig. 3–24A). The off-set pin should not catch on the edge of the FC pin but should have good support (Fig. 3–24B). The amount of exposure of the top surface of the FC pin will determine the amount of freedom in centric in the anteroposterior movement from centric occlusion to centric relation, and laterally in relation to the degree to which the lateral wings are raised. Note the relationship in Figure 3–25A,B,C.

When a lateral wing is elevated slightly and the upper member of the articulator moved into lateral (right working), the off-set pin makes contact with the table (Fig. 3–26A). The contact occurs even more quickly as the wing is raised farther.

Freedom in Centric (Lateral)

The magnitude of the freedom in centric that may be obtained on the H2 articulator using the Schuyler pin and table will depend to an extent on the settings of the wings and table required for guidance. Since the lateral wings and incisal guide table inclination are predetermined, the magnitude of the lateral freedom in centric will be related to the length of freedom in centric. The influence of the pin varies

Text continued on page 63

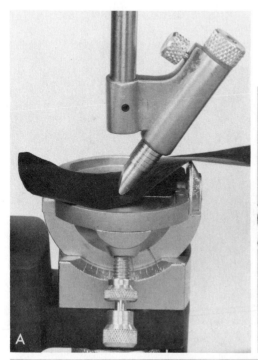

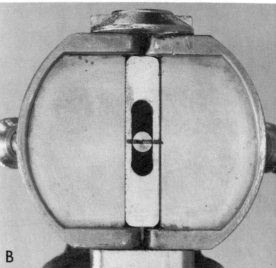

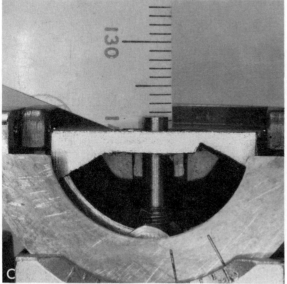

Figure 3–21. Setting the incisal guide and FC pin. *A*, Use of articulating paper to mark contact of incisal pin on table; *B*, off-set pin has been centered; *C*, raise FC pin in relation to necessary inclination of the incisal table.

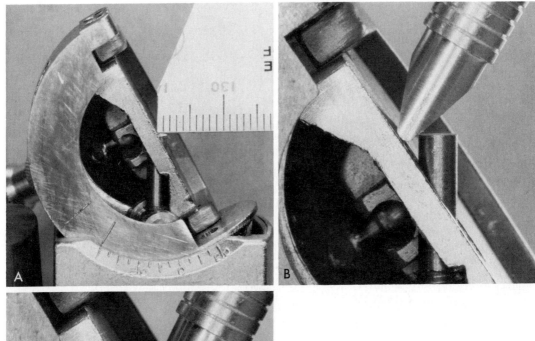

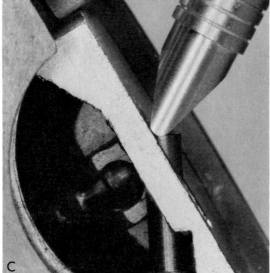

Figure 3–22. Setting incisal guide and FC pin. *A*, FC pin is elevated in relation to incisal table inclination to provide the amount of freedom in centric required. *B*, FC pin elevated too much; *C*, correct elevation.

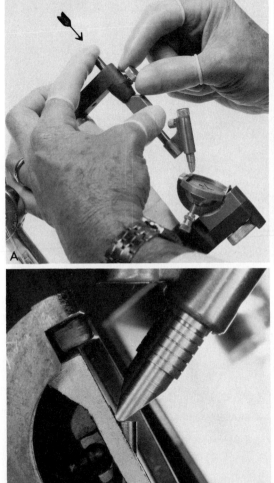

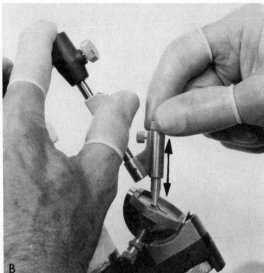

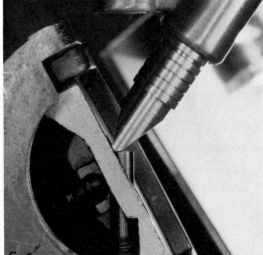

Figure 3–23. Setting incisal pin and table. Simultaneous adjustment of central pin and off-set pin (see text).

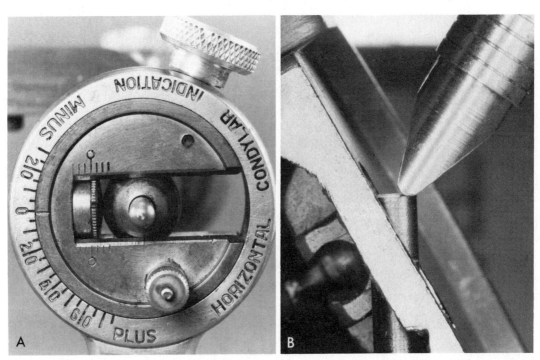

Figure 3–24. Setting incisal pin and table. *A*, condylar element against centric stop with casts in centric relation position; *B*, off-set pin touching anterior part of FC pin. Contact should be present at centric occlusion and centric relation if the occlusal adjustment has been done correctly.

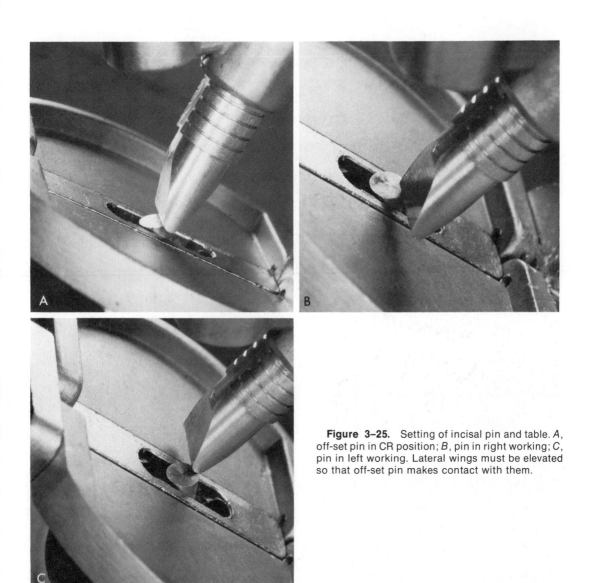

Figure 3–25. Setting of incisal pin and table. *A*, off-set pin in CR position; *B*, pin in right working; *C*, pin in left working. Lateral wings must be elevated so that off-set pin makes contact with them.

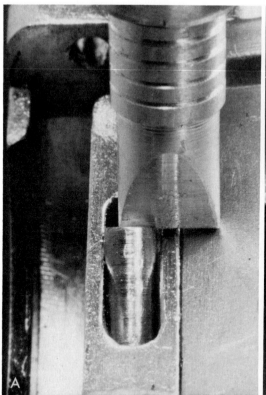
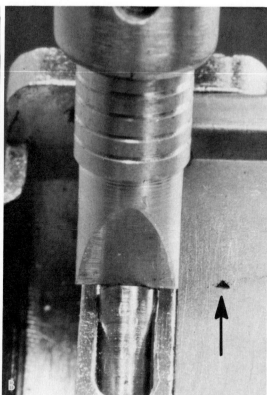
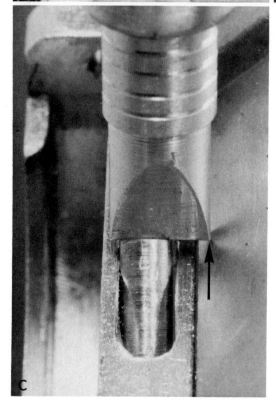

Figure 3–26. Setting lateral wings of incisal table. *A*, contact of edge of off-set pin with slight elevation of left wing; *B*, arrow and point shows point of contact; *C*, with greater elevation of the wing contact is made with slight lateral movement (pin in centric relation position).

Table 3–1 Length vs. Width of Freedom in Centric (Schuyler Pin and Table)

DISTANCE OF PIN FROM CR	ANGULATION OF		FC WIDTH
	WINGS	INCISAL TABLE	
Centric relation	20	30	2 mm
0.5 mm	20	30	1.5 mm
1.0 mm	20	30	1 mm
1.5 mm	20	30	0.5 mm
Centric occlusion	20	30	.25 mm

with centric relation and centric occlusion, the width of freedom in centric being greater at centric relation than at centric occlusion. The movement from centric occlusion to centric relation and between is required for freedom in centric on the articulator. A brief table (Table 3–1) shows the type of relationship that can exist between the width and the length of freedom in centric. The table is for projections on a frontal plane passing between the first molars.

These numbers are relative inasmuch as the angulation of the wings or the incisal table or both will influence the width of freedom in centric. The general approach is to consider this: the closer the incisal table is to the incisal pin, the less the freedom in centric width will be. In effect, the greater the centric occlusion to centric relation distance dictated by the central FC pin of the incisal table, the greater the width of freedom in centric (other factors remaining constant).

The higher the incisal table and the lateral wings, the closer the incisal table is to the off-set incisal pin. However, the freedom in centric may be increased or decreased on the articulator for various reasons, and it is possible to obtain a variety of combinations of lateral wing angulation, incisal table angulation, and centric occlusion–centric relation distance that give about the same lateral freedom in centric width. If, however, the wings, table, and centric occlusion–centric relation distance are all at predetermined loca-tions or cannot or should not be changed, the freedom in centric width follows as a consequence of the predetermined set-tings.

From a practical standpoint, the dif-ference in lateral freedom in centric between centric relation and centric occlu-sion is greatest with the greatest antero-posterior freedom in centric. Probably a right and left lateral freedom of 1 mm is adequate in most instances. The practical limits of the Schuyler pin and table would appear to be about 2 mm freedom in cen-tric. With the table at 60° and the lateral wings at 40° and a centric occlusion to centric relation distance of 1 mm at the condylar elements, there is a 1 mm lateral freedom in centric at centric relation, and about .5 mm at centric occlusion. In most instances, the difference between centric occlusion and centric relation is about .25 to .5 mm.

The shape of the freedom in centric produced by the Schuyler pin and table at the molar (projection to the horizontal plane) is more like a triangle than an ovoid or a circle. The difference in width be-tween centric occlusion and centric rela-tion also contributes to the variation in shapes produced by the off-set pin on the central FC pin of the incisal table. No doubt, the shape of the blade of the off-set pin also influences the final form of the freedom in centric. These variations in form have no bearing on the final function except when the freedom in centric area may be inadequate in size.

Unit 3 Exercises

1. The anteroposterior steepness of the incisal guide table is determined by

   _____ .

2. If all maxillary anterior teeth are absent, how is the incisal guide table set?

   _____

3. What are the functions of the incisal guide pin and table?

   _____

4. When is a customized incisal guidance used?

   _____

5. How is freedom in centric obtained with the Schuyler pin and table?

   _____

6. In order to use a Schuyler system on articulated casts for the purpose of waxing multiple restorations (less than full mouth reconstruction), why is it necessary to do an occlusal adjustment to freedom in centric on the patient?

   _____

   _____

7. When should an occlusal adjustment be done?

   _____

8. A patient has an occlusal interference in centric relation but no functional disturbances. Inasmuch as no occlusal adjustment is indicated under the circumstances, what is done about freedom in centric for a single restoration?

   _____

   _____

9. When an occlusal adjustment has been done for a patient and a 1 mm freedom in centric has been established in the natural dentition, what should be the dimensions of freedon in centric in a single full crown restoration?

   _____

   _____

10. To what extent should freedom in centric be developed in a three-unit bridge when a lateral slide in centric has been eliminated in the natural dentition by an occlusal adjustment?

   _____

Unit 3 Test

1. The steepness of incisal guidance is:

   a. not important for neuromuscular harmony
   b. unrelated to vertical overlap
   c. a and b
   d. simulated on the Hanau incisal table by the lateral wings
   e. a, b, and d

2. In the absence of maxillary incisors, the incisal guide table is set by:

   a. posterior teeth
   b. inclination of condylar guidance
   c. cuspid guidance when possible
   d. slide in centric
   e. position of centric occlusion

3. Which of the following is not a function of an adjustable pin and table:

   a. to maintain vertical dimension
   b. to prevent wearing down of stone casts
   c. to indicate the extent to which occlusal contact relations should be waxed
      in a restoration
   d. to facilitate an increased vertical dimension
   e. no exceptions

4. An incisal guide is customized to:

   a. increase incisal steepness if necessary
   b. allow for curvatures in movement paths
   c. a and b
   d. allow greater influence by condylar guidance
   e. a, b, and d

5. The Schuyler pin and table:

   a. allows for flat inclined plane guidance
   b. provides for flat horizontal plane guidance
   c. a and b
   d. provides curved inclined plane guidance
   e. a, b, and d

6. A Schuyler pin and table can be used for:

   a. single restorations
   b. multiple restorations
   c. full mouth reconstruction
   d. complete dentures
   e. all of the above

7. In the absence of freedom in centric on casts:

   a. a Schuyler pin and table need not be used
   b. the FC pin should be below the surface of the incisal table
   c. a and b
   d. a straight incisal pin can be used if vertical dimension is not to be
      changed
   e. a, b, and d

8. After elimination of premature contacts in centric relation by an occlusal adjustment, the freedom in centric is 1 mm. In waxing a restoration on an articulator using a Schuyler pin and table, the freedom in centric should be:

    a. 0.5 mm
    b. 1.0 mm
    c. 1.5 mm
    d. 2.0 mm
    e. none of the above

9. The lateral dimension of freedom in centric will depend upon:

    a. extent of lateral slide in centric
    b. anteroposterior steepness of incisal table
    c. a and b
    d. steepness of inclination of lateral wings
    e. a, b, and d

10. Vertical dimension may be maintained by an incisal pin that:

    a. is curved with a radius related to the axis of the articulator
    b. has an off-set pin related to the arc of closure of the upper member of the articulator
    c. a and b
    d. can be adjusted in length
    e. a, b, and d

Unit 4

Face Bow: Parts and Function

The face bow, its use, and its functional parts are discussed here; its application in the mounting of casts on an articulator is demonstrated in Unit 7. Two basic types of simple face bows are in general use: an ear piece and a non ear piece face bow. In both, an arbitrary method is used for determining the hinge axis of the mandible. In order to determine the true hinge axis, a kinematic face bow or hinge axis locator is used.

This unit is concerned with the theory of the simple face bow and the transfer of the relationship between the condyles and the maxillary arch to the articulator. The details of the use of the face bow in the mounting of casts are found in Unit 7.

INTRODUCTION: UNIT OBJECTIVES AND READINGS

The objectives of this unit relate to the face bow and its function. Several behavioral objectives are suggested.
A. Objectives
   1. Be able to identify:
      a. components of a simple face bow
      b. the arbitrary hinge axis.
   2. Be able to differentiate between a simple face bow and a kinematic face bow.
B. Reading
   Brandrup-Wognoson, T.: The face bow: Its significance and application. J. Prosthet. Dent. 3:618, 1953.

DEFINITIONS

The face bow has been identified as "a device which serves the purpose of meas-uring the positional relationship of the maxillary ridge and teeth to the middle of the glenoid fossa in three dimensions, namely sagittal, vertical, and anterior-posterior."[1] Hanau identifies the face bow as an instrument that records the correct positional relation of the maxillary ridge and teeth in the patient and transfers this relation to the articulator, thereby producing a positional relation, which enhances succinct interpretation of maxillomandibular conditions.[2]

From these definitions some indication of the face bow's function is given. Why is it necessary to have a common frame of reference between the patient and the articulator? It is necessary in order to have a meaningful positional relationship of the casts on the articulator that is close to, if not identical with in a practical sense, that relationship found between the maxilla and mandible (including the condyles).

Another approach to understanding the significance of the face bow is to consider what would be done without a face bow and the effect on occlusal relations. Before the time of Gysi there was no instrument for finding or recording centric relation. Gysi's approach to maxillomandibular relations was the "Gothic Arch" tracing (see Fig. 1–5). In 1899, Snow developed a face bow to position casts of edentulous mouths on an articulator. Gysi, who recognized the inexactness of the method, located the "hinge axis" by palpating the joints. By

---

[1]J. S. Landa: Practical Full Denture Prosthesis, 2nd edition. Brooklyn, N.Y., Dental Items of Interest Publishing Co., 1954.

[2]R. L. Hanau: Full Denture Prosthesis: Intratechnique for Hanau Articulator Model H, 4th edition. Buffalo, N.Y., privately printed, 1940, p. 12.

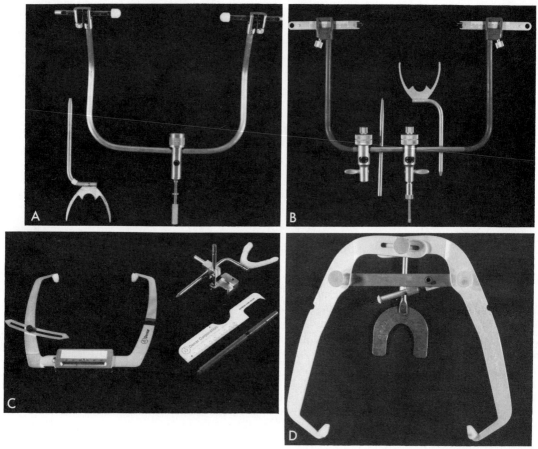

Figure 4–1. Face bow. Manually centered face bows: *A*, Hanau; *B*, Dentatus. Self-centering face bows: *C*, Denar; *D*, Whip-mix.

Parts of the Face Bow
Figure 4-4

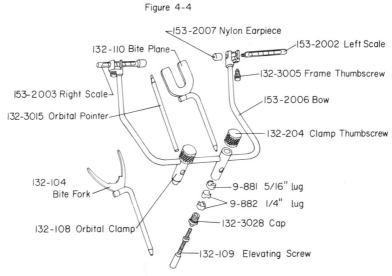

153-2007 Nylon Earpiece
132-110 Bite Plane
153-2002 Left Scale
132-3005 Frame Thumbscrew
153-2003 Right Scale
153-2006 Bow
132-3015 Orbital Pointer
132-204 Clamp Thumbscrew
132-104 Bite Fork
9-881 5/16" Lug
9-882 1/4" Lug
132-108 Orbital Clamp
132-3028 Cap
132-109 Elevating Screw

Figure 4–2. Parts of the Hanau ear piece face bow.

using the face bow to describe maxillo-condylar relations and the "Gothic Arch" tracing to describe maxillomandibular relations, Gysi was able to use a semi-adjustable articulator with some effectiveness.

PARTS OF A FACE BOW

Most adjustable and semi-adjustable articulators have some type of face bow as accessory equipment. Two types of ear piece face bows are available: (1) manually centered and (2) self-centering. The Hanau (Fig. 4–1A) is an ear piece manual centering device; the Dentatus (Fig. 4–1B) is a manual centering type that requires measurement of the hinge axis; the Denar (Fig. 4–1C) and the Whip-Mix (Fig. 4–1D) are self-centering ear piece face bows. The parts of the Hanau are fully identified in Figure 4–2. A brief overview of the use of the face bow transfer follows.

A QUICK LOOK AT USE OF THE FACE BOW

1. Base plate wax is softened into a roll and placed on a bite plane. While the wax is soft, place the bite plane into the mouth and press into position on the maxillary teeth (Fig. 4–3A).

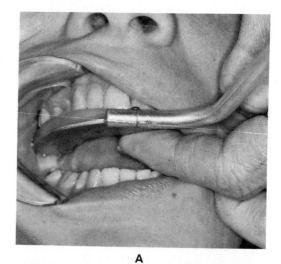

A

2. Remove the bite plane and chill the wax. Indentations should appear in the wax, but the metal frame should not be touched by the teeth (Fig. 4–3B).

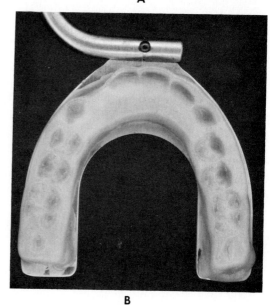

B

3. Relate the face bow to the patient's arbitrary hinge axis automatically with the ear piece face bow (Fig. 4–4) or by use of the non ear piece face bow and measurement (Fig. 4–5).

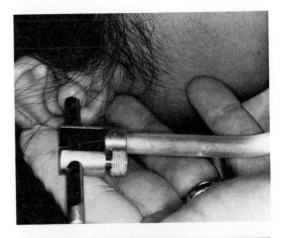

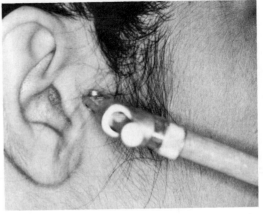

4. Lock the face bow in position on the bite plane when the face bow is centered (Fig. 4–6) and transfer to the articulator.

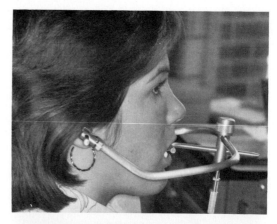

5. The face bow is centered on the articulator and the bite plane raised to the third reference point on the incisal pin (Fig. 4–7). Attach the maxillary cast to the mounting ring with impression plaster.

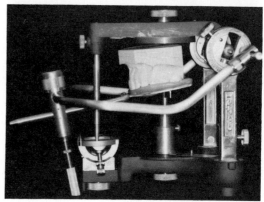

ANALYSIS OF FACE BOW PROCEDURE

The maxillary dentition has a three-dimensional relationship to all condylar movement. Deviation from this relationship causes change in the resultant movement of the mandibular dentition over the maxillary dentition. There are several possible reasons why deviation may occur when the actual state of the patient's mouth is compared to his mounted stone casts on the articulator.

When the face bow is not used to relate the maxillary cast to the approximated starting positions of the condyles, the resulting arcs of movement may differ from the patient to the articulator. This lack of coincidence may cause restorations fabricated on the articulator to have potential occlusal errors.

Visualize fabricating a cusped tooth restoration with the working casts in the incorrect position.

1. Could the restoration be an occlusal interference in the opening and closing movement? Describe briefly.

_____

_____

2. Could the restoration be an occlusal interference in lateral or lateroprotrusive excursion? Describe briefly.

_____

_____

3. Observe other mountings. Is there any variation indicating patient differences?

_____

_____

4. If the maxillary arch is asymmetrically positioned in relation to the skull, should the face bow transfer to the articulator reflect this?

_____

_____

Two essential steps are utilized to orient the maxillary cast on the articulator. First, the transverse hinge must be located by average anatomic measurement (average, semi-adjustable articulators) or kinematically (fully adjustable articulators); second, the orientation of the occlusal plane is determined by selecting some arbitrary anterior point of reference such as a notch on the incisal pin.

The third point of reference with the transverse axis forms a horizontal plane of reference. Some techniques may utilize other landmarks (Fig. 4–8) such as the infraorbital point or 43 mm superior to the edge of the maxillary incisor. Using different planes and points for the third reference results in raising or lowering the anterior portion of the face bow, and eventually the maxillary cast in the articulator.

The simple face bow, but not the ear piece type, raises and lowers about a fixed radius and as it raises it appears to move slightly forward. Figure 4–9 depicts the occlusal plane and corresponding projected condylar inclinations for the same case mounted with various third points of reference. The anteroposterior difference in the position of the cast appears to produce minimal error if the upward/downward position does not exceed ± 16 mm. Note that the Hanau ear piece face bow does not directly couple with the axis of the articulator (Fig. 4–10). This special problem is discussed in Unit 8.

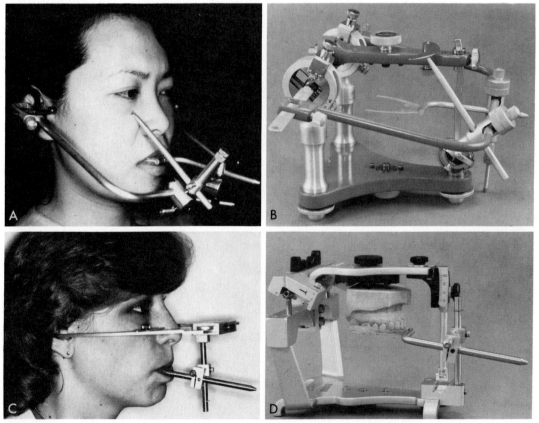

Figure 4–8. Third point of reference for face bow transfer. *A,* infraorbital pointer; *B,* orientation of pointer to articulator; *C,* point of reference 43 mm superior to edge of incisor; *D,* orientation of point to the articulator.

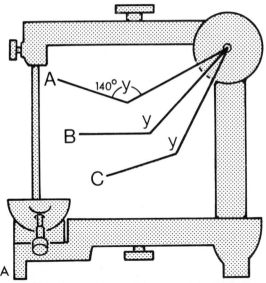

Figure 4–9. Effect of position of third point of reference on anteroposterior position of the maxillary cast. *A,* The relationship of face bow and occlusal plane remains fixed (Angle Y) but as the third point is elevated or lowered, the anteroposterior position of the cast is changed; *B,* maxillary cast elevated; *C,* cast lowered. Note change in anteroposterior position of incisal edges of teeth.

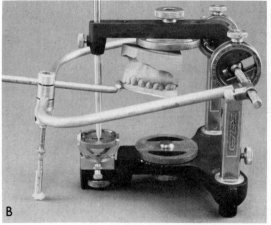

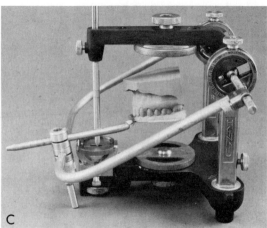

Figure 4–10. Ear piece face bow and third point of reference. Third point of reference is fixed at ~58 mm because ear piece does not attach to axis of the articulator.

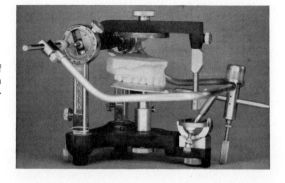

Unit 4 Exercises

1. What effect does raising or lowering the face bow have on the ultimate centric occlusion?

2. What effect does raising the third point of reference have on horizontal condylar inclination?

3. According to one author, if the horizontal condylar inclination is changed from 40° to 31° and the incisal guidance is unchanged in relation to the occlusal plane, the effect seen in the molar area on the balancing side of identical casts mounted utilizing third points of reference 26 mm apart would be:

4. What are the limitations set by the horizontal condylar guidance of the articulator in raising or lowering the face bow?

5. What is the purpose in raising the face bow so the incisal edges of the maxillary incisors approximate the notch on the incisal pin of the Hanau H2–PR articulator (non ear piece type).

6. What is the basis for the ear pieces on a simple face bow?

7. If the maxillary arch is asymmetrically positioned in relation to the skull, should the face bow transfer to the articulator reflect this?

8. What is the average error in finding the true hinge axis using a simple face bow? Using a kinematic face bow or hinge axis locator?

_____

_____

_____

9. What is the value of using a third point of reference in mounting casts with the face bow?

_____

_____

10. If a maxillary cast is not centered on the articulator, and the transfer has been made correctly, does this present a problem?

_____

_____

11. What may be the extent of the error in not using a face bow, i.e., mounting the maxillary cast in the center of the articulator with the occlusal plane parallel to the base of the articulator (using a non ear piece face bow)?

_____

_____

12. If the cast is mounted in the center of the articulator without a face bow, how may the potential errors be minimized?

_____

_____

Unit 4 Test

1. A simple (Snow) face bow is used to:

   a. mount the mandibular cast in relation to the maxillary cast
   b. relate the maxilla to a transverse axis of the temporomandibular joints
   c. relate the maxillary dentition to the infraorbital notch
   d. relate the maxillary cast to the transverse axis of the articulators so that the axle axis and the true hinge axis are coincident
   e. all of the above

2. The error of using a simple face bow rather than a kinematic face bow:

   a. is about 0.2 mm anteroposteriorly if the CR wax bite is 5 to 10 mm thick
   b. may not be clinically significant if the CR check bite is less than 0.5 mm thick
   c. is nonexistent if the mandibular registration is made at "CO = CR"
   d. is greater when the face bow is not self-centering
   e. none of the above

3. With a properly mounted cast on an adequate articulator:

   a. centric occlusion and centric relation contacts should be the same as intraoral contacts
   b. an opening between posterior centric stops (supporting cusps and fossae) is not permissible
   c. all tooth contacts in centric occlusion that occur in the mouth should occur on the casts
   d. balancing side contacts should be present if present in the mouth
   e. all of the above

4. Concerning the "true" hinge axis, it is obtained by:

   a. the kinematic face bow
   b. CR registration bite
   c. simple face bow
   d. an ear piece type face bow
   e. all of the above

5. The simple face bow:

   a. locates the terminal hinge axis
   b. is taken in centric relation
   c. relates the mandible to the hinge axis
   d. may be a non ear piece device
   e. none of the above

6. An orbital clamp and pointer on the simple face bow is used:

   a. to relate the maxillary cast to an infraorbital point
   b. to locate a third point of reference for mounting the maxillary cast
   c. a and b
   d. only with an ear piece face bow
   e. a, b, and d

7. The points of reference for a simple non ear piece:

   a. arbitrary hinge axis and notch on incisal pin
   b. arbitrary hinge axis and infraorbital point
   c. a and b
   d. true hinge axis and upper notch on incisal pin
   e. a, b, and d

8. A simple face bow:

   a. is not centered on the head
   b. with ear pieces is not centered on the axis of the articulator
   c. a and b
   d. is centered on the articulator
   e. a, b, and d

9. All of the following may be restorative errors related to not using a face bow or to its incorrect use in mounting the maxillary cast on an articulator except:

    a. anteroposterior error in occlusal morphology

    b. lateral error in placement of cusps and fossae

    c. incorrect relationship of control between condylar and incisal guidances of articulator

    d. improper contact relations of wear facets on casts in lateral excursions

    e. no exceptions

10. If a face bow is not used on the H2–PR articulator, how may some of errors introduced in waxing of restorations be minimized?

    a. make occlusal plane as parallel to condylar inclination as reasonably possible

    b. maximize tooth guidance in various positions by changing condylar guidance for the positions

    c. a and b

    d. provide for freedom in centric

    e. a, b, and d

Unit 5

Simple Articulators

A simple hinge-like device is often used for relating casts of the occlusal surfaces of several opposing teeth in order to make an individual restoration or multiple restorations. Even when the device (or articulator, as it may be incorrectly called) has some provision for vertical and horizontal movement, errors in occlusal morphology are likely to occur. Even when the errors are recognized and minimized in the restoration on the simple "articulator," some untoward responses of the masticatory system to the residual error may not be eliminated, even with the patient in the dental chair. Such an approach is not practical or desirable for multiple or complex restorations. Furthermore, it is not efficient to take a lot of chair time to "grind in" restorations. Besides the inefficiency, the loss of occlusal margins and functional anatomy does not suggest that the best treatment has been provided to the patient. However, very fine treatment may be rendered if the clinician limits the use of the simple "articulator" to those individual restorations in which he is able to anticipate errors, avoid them, and provide treatment efficiently. Efficient treatment by definition is effective and of high quality. An efficient clinician knows his own limitations and the limitations of the instruments he uses, and is able to adjust to these limitations.

INTRODUCTION: UNIT OBJECTIVES AND READINGS

Unit 5 will serve as only a brief introduction to some of the limitations of, or errors resulting from the use of, simple articulator devices in dental treatment, especially restorations with major involvement of the occlusal surface. Because the unit is introductory, the objectives are limited in scope and require behavioral responses

that are concerned principally with discovering how occlusal interferences may develop from the use of a simple Class II nonadjustable articulator or straight line articulator. Several behavioral objectives are considered.

A. Objectives
 1. Be able to identify the major errors in occlusion that can result from using a simple nonadjustable articulator.
 2. Be able to indicate methods for reducing the errors in occlusion that result from using a simple nonadjustable articulator.
 3. Be able to provide a rational alternative when the error of using a simple nonadjustable articulator cannot be eliminated entirely.
B. Readings (optional)
 McPhee, E. R.: The simple class II nonadjustable articulator: Limitations, errors, and compensating procedures. J. Michigan Dent. Assn. 56:68–73, 1974.
 Celenza, Frank V.: Articulators and determinants of occlusal morphology. Articulators. *In* International Prosthodontic Workshop (on Complete Denture Occlusion), Lang, B. R. and Kelsey, C. C., Eds. University of Michigan, 1973, pp. 90–92.

LIMITATIONS OF SIMPLE ARTICULATORS

A number of questions arise concerning the use of the simple* type of articulator (Fig. 5–1). Most relate to problems arising from the size of the articulator and the interocclusal record used to mount the

---

*For example, an instrument that permits horizontal as well as vertical motion, but not related to the motion of the temporomandibular joints.

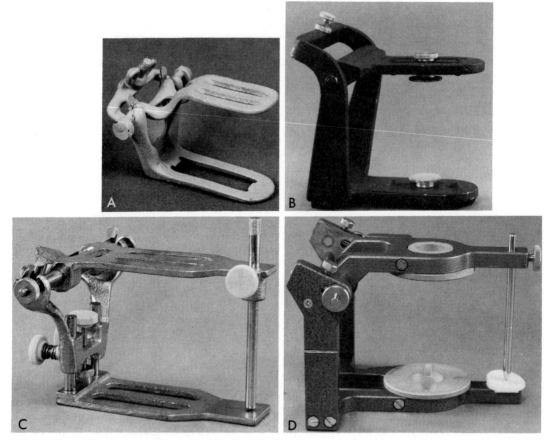

Figure 5–1. Simple articulators. *A* to *D*, articulators increasing in size from small to normal size and with varying kinds of convenience but nonfunctional adjustments.

casts of segments of arches in the articulator.

What are the major limitations of a simple articulator?

The contact occlusal relationships in eccentric movements are unrelated to the patient; there is no provision for movement into centric relation; the centric occlusion position may not be accurately defined (freedom in centric).

Which errors may occur from the limitations of a simple articulator?

Included are premature contacts in centric occlusion, centric relation, balancing interferences, protrusive and working interferences.

Interocclusal Registration (Centric Occlusion)

After a tooth has been prepared (cavity preparation) and a dental restoration is to be made away from the dental chair, impressions are made of the teeth having the cavity preparation and the opposing teeth. These impressions are poured in stone and must be articulated (occlusal surfaces related). Consider that errors in tooth position may already have been introduced because of shifting of the teeth. The stone casts often involve only half a mouth or less, and the simple articulator frame not much more than a straight line. In order to attach the maxillary and mandibular casts to the upper and lower frames, some type of interocclusal registration ("wax bite") is frequently used. The interocclusal registration in centric occlusion is not necessarily registering centric occlusion and is almost always a major source of articulation error.

Why is the interocclusal registration of centric occlusion a frequent major source of occlusal error?

Because the hinge axis of the articulator is not the same as that of the patient.

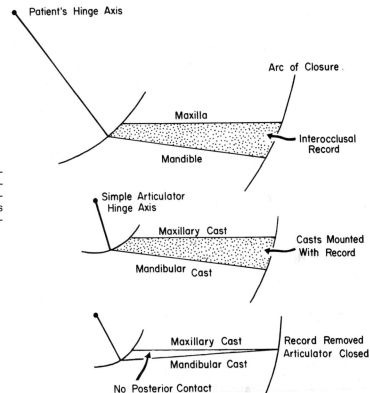

Figure 5–2. Schematic representation of the effect of articulator size on the relationship between the patient's hinge axis and the axis of the small articulator.

Consequently *any* thickness to the interocclusal record will result in an incorrect relationship between the maxillary and mandibular casts. A *zero* thickness *interocclusal* record (check bite in centric) is not possible and some error will invariably be present.

How does the difference in location of the transverse hinge axis between the patient and the simple articulator cause error when the interocclusal record has thickness?

The arcs of closure for the patient's mandible and the upper member of the articulator are different (Fig. 5–2). For consistency the lower member of the articulator is shown being closed. Figure 5–3 shows the effect of any thickness of the check bite on contact vertical dimension when a small simple articulator is used.

What is the error that occurs from using a simple articulator and an interocclusal record with thickness?

A posterior restoration would be made to

Figure 5–3. Schematic representation of the effect of an interocclusal record (wax check bite) of centric occlusion when using a small articulator. *A,* difference in location of patient's hinge axis and hinge axis of articulator; *B,* after check bite is removed, note absence of posterior contacts in centric occlusion.

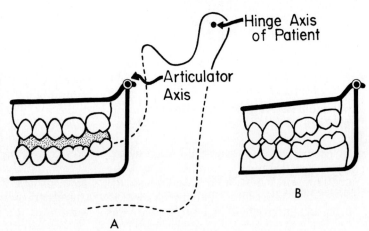

contact when the articulator was closed (anterior contact only) but would be "high" when placed in the mouth. This error requires grinding of the restoration to allow complete closure, often resulting in loss of the margins of a restoration on the occlusal surface. The error always degrades the surface characteristics and functional morphology.

How is the error of the simple articulator and interocclusal record avoided?

There are two obvious solutions: (1) Do not use a simple type articulator; use a full-size articulator and a centric relation interocclusal record. (2) Do not use an interocclusal record (check bite) with a simple articulator. Although the first solution is preferred, it may not be practical or realistic for individual restorations; the second is the practical solution.

How are casts articulated on a simple articulator without using an interocclusal record?

There are two solutions: (1) Take full arch impressions and position the casts in centric occlusion for mounting, or (2) have the patient close into centric occlusion and take a lateral record of the facial surfaces of the teeth. The record should be small in size. Impression plaster, compound, or wax should be used. Half-arch or less casts can be positioned in centric occlusion in the lateral record and mounted in the simple articulator.

Are there any other sources of error from using a simple articulator?

Inasmuch as the casts are mounted in centric occlusion (the articulator has no provision for use of a CR check bite method), there is no possibility of moving into centric relation and no possibility of using a simulated centric relation even if a simulated centric relation were a valid technique.

Interocclusal Registration (Centric Relation)

A centric relation interocclusal registration record cannot be used to mount the maxillary and mandibular casts in a small-size simple articulator. The arc of closure on the articulator will not be the same as that which occurs on the patient and the initial point of occlusal contact will be different. In effect, the centric relation contact will be different on the articulator from that in the patient, and cusp tips and fossae may be placed in a position in a restoration being made on a simple articulator that will be incorrect when the restoration is placed in the mouth. Furthermore, the height and depth of cusps and fossae will be incorrect for posterior teeth for the same reasons given for the error when mounting in centric occlusion.

In addition to the anteroposterior error and vertical error (height of cusp and fossa), the simple articulator may have no provision for anterior movement to glide from centric relation to centric occlusion when the casts have been mounted in centric relation. This limitation of the articulator is contrary to making restorations with freedom in centric.

Size of Articulator

Why not use a full-size simple articulator to avoid anteroposterior and vertical errors?

There are simple articulators that have dimensions that are equivalent on the average to a patient and to an articulator such as the Hanau H2–PR. Such articulators tend to reduce anteroposterior and vertical errors greatly, especially vertical errors, unlike the simple small articulator. However, further reductions require the use of a face bow (arbitrary hinge axis location) or the use of a kinematic face bow or true hinge axis locator. This procedure requires more instrumentation as well as operator skill in obtaining a centric relation registration. Very rapidly the articulator and mounting procedure become more than a simple articulator and procedure.

The question is asked of whether it is practical and necessary to go beyond the simple small articulator for individual restorations. The question is related to large and small articulators.

If a large simple articulator is more accurate to use than a small simple articulator, why not use the large articulator?

Indeed, why not? The answer is not as ·simple as it appears. The large articulator is not used because it is large. It takes up more space; it cannot as easily be mailed, carried, or stored as the small articulator. In the technician's laboratory, a full-size articulator takes up more bench space and is harder to grasp. It is more difficult to see around and is more expensive. Even having 15 to 20 small articulators around during various stages of dental procedures puts a strain on space and inventory costs. Unfortunately, the simple small articulator has no provision for transferring casts to different articulators. It takes a very well made and special instrument to be able to use a set of casts on different articulators. To do so means that the articulator is no longer simple. Finally, more plaster is needed to mount the casts — more weight, more expense to mail, and so forth. In short, the large articulator may not be practical except when the dentist has his own laboratory at the office or does his own individual restorations. How the size of the articulator relates to centric relation or centric occlusion is a question that is appropriate at this point.

For single or individual restorations of a molar is it better (less error) to use: (1) a full-size simple articulator, full arch casts and no interocclusal record for centric occlusion; (2) a full-size simple articulator, full arch casts, and a centric relation interocclusal record; (3) a full-size simple articulator, full arch casts, and a centric occlusion interocclusal record; or (4) a small simple articulator, less than full arch casts, and a lateral occlusal registration for centric occlusion to mount the casts?

The answer is 1 when considering the least error, but 4 is the most practical method of dealing with individual restorations. However, the most rational method is to use a modest size simple articulator, full arch casts when possible, and no interocclusal registration record (casts articulated in centric occlusion) for mounting the casts. At this point the design of the restoration is dependent on anticipated lateral and protrusive movements and the location of centric relation contact position.

What are the most common restorative errors made with a simple articulator?

By far the most common errors are: (1)

premature contacts in centric relation on the oblique ridge of maxillary molars and the mesial cusp ridge of the lingual cusp of the maxillary first premolar; (2) balancing interference involving the lingual cusps of the maxillary first molar; (3) working side interference involving mandibular and maxillary buccal cusps and lingual cusps, i.e., axial surfaces of lingual cusps of the maxillary molars; and (4) premature contacts in centric occlusion involving the posterior teeth. Almost all occur at some time, but the last one listed (premature contact in centric occlusion) is often the only one easily noticed by the clinician and patient — at least when the restoration is first placed in the mouth. The masticatory system may adapt to the others to varying degrees. The minimization of premature contacts in centric occlusion has already been suggested.

How are premature contacts in centric relation minimized on the small articulator?

This is accomplished by moving the oblique ridge distally and reducing its height and by reducing the height of the mesial cusp ridge of the lingual cusp of the maxillary first premolar as well as moving it distally.

Eccentric Movements

The relationship between eccentric movements and the size or similarity of the articulator is obvious from a hypothetical point of view when the "condylar determinants of occlusion" are considered. However, the errors related to lateral shift, intercondylar distance, and other such measures are not so gross or obvious as those errors that arise because of a failure to consider the tooth determinants of occlusion. There are several questions that must be considered in relating occlusal determinants to eccentric movements. Most simple articulators have no provisions for condylar guidance adjustment. They have a fixed condylar element path for lateral and protrusive movements, but the path has no relationship to the patient nor can it be changed to relate to occlusal contacts or facets of wear present on the casts. However, the answers to a few questions may provide some guidance in making restorations on a simple articulator.

What determines the height and overlap of buccal cusps for working positions?

The presence or absence of cuspid guidance and posterior contacts on the patient (determined from observation of the patient when impressions and history are taken or "read" from facets of wear on casts). The height, overlap, and contact of buccal cusps must be consistent with adjacent cusps. Final grinding must be done in the mouth. A wax "chew-in" from the patient is most helpful when using a small articulator with limited eccentric movement.

What determines the height and form of the lingual cusps in balancing position if tooth guidance cannot be related to the articulator?

There are only one or two articulators which provide that the occlusion (contacting tooth surfaces) determines the movements of the condylar elements. They are full-size instruments. Thus the relationship of the lingual cusp of the maxillary molar to the buccal cusp in balancing must be determined by relating it to the patient or facets of wear (or lack of them) on the casts. A general principle for the lingual cusps of the maxillary posterior teeth can be formulated in terms of the following question.

How is the error of balancing interferences minimized when using a simple articulator?

Make certain the preparation involving reduction of occlusal surfaces is adequate. For molar preparations reduce all mesial and distal cusp ridges of lingual cusps on maxillary teeth, or all mesial and distal cusp ridges of buccal cusps of mandibular molars. Know the paths that cusps follow on opposing teeth.

What other errors must be minimized with the simple articulator?

Interferences involving the axial surfaces of maxillary molars and the buccal slopes of the lingual cusps of mandibular molars are areas that must not be overcontoured because they will then be working interferences.

Unit 5 Exercises

1. Name the error introduced by using an interocclusal record in a small simple type of articulator.

   _____

2. The error introduced by an interocclusal record when using a small simple type articulator will result in a posterior restoration that is _____ .

3. A centric relation check bite (is, is not) useful for mounting complete or partial casts on a small simple type articulator.

4. List a practical solution to minimizing errors introduced by an interocclusal record.

   _____

5. How can working and balancing interferences be minimized when waxing a restoration on a small simple articulator?

   _____

6. Is it possible to precisely prevent all errors in a restoration that has been waxed on a small simple articulator? Why?

   _____

   _____

7. What errors may be reduced by using a full-sized simple articulator?

   _____

   _____

8. For a single individual restoration of a molar, what is the best way to prevent errors in the occlusion?

   _____

9. Why not use a full-sized articulator for all restorative dentistry?

   _____

10. If a patient has molar group function and a maxillary first molar full crown restoration is being waxed, how can buccal cusps be formed when using a simple type articulator which has no possibility for lateral movements?

    _____

Unit 5 Test

1. A simple articulator:

   a. may permit horizontal movement
   b. does permit vertical movement
   c. a and b
   d. is related to the motion of the temporomandibular joints
   e. a, b, and d

2. When using a small simple articulator, contact vertical dimension error in the molar area would be minimized if the centric occlusion check bite:

   a. has zero thickness
   b. is made of very soft wax
   c. is taken in centric relation
   d. is taken in centric occlusion
   e. none of the above

3. A thick centric occlusion check bite could result in a molar restoration having:

   a. premature contact in centric occlusion when placed in the mouth
   b. absence of centric stops
   c. lateral interferences
   d. protrusive interferences
   e. all of the above

4. In order to avoid errors in contact vertical dimension on molar restorations, it is necessary to:

   a. use full arch casts
   b. not use an interocclusal record
   c. a and b
   d. use a full-size articulator
   e. a, b, and d

5. A functionally generated path (or wax chew-in) technique may be used to:

   a. minimize errors in waxing eccentric occlusal contacts
   b. avoid all errors in contact vertical dimension
   c. a and b
   d. avoid all anteroposterior errors in the occlusion of individual restorations
   e. a, b, and d

6. When an anterior maxillary crown or bridge is made, the use of a simple type of articulator with no provisions for lateral or protrusive movements will result usually in:

   a. excessive grinding on the restorations in the mouth
   b. protrusive interferences
   c. a and b
   d. premature contact in centric relation
   e. a, b, and d

7. Compared with a "small-size" articulator the use of a "large-size" articulator for individual restorations:

    a. gives the best results
    b. is often not practical
    c. a and b
    d. is always indicated
    e. a, b, and d

8. Which of the following is likely to lead to the fewest errors when using a small simple articulator having capability for some lateral movements:

    a. molar group function
    b. cuspid guidance only
    c. balanced occlusion
    d. anterior open bite
    e. 2 mm discrepancy between centric occlusion and centric relation

9. The mounting of full arch casts on a small simple articulator:

    a. is not practical when posterior teeth are absent
    b. without a check bite decreases potential vertical errors in restorations
    c. a and b
    d. will eliminate premature contacts in centric relation for molar restorations
    e. a, b, and d

10. When simple articulators are used, occlusal interferences may be minimized on restorations by:

    a. moving oblique ridges distally
    b. reducing the axial contours of maxillary lingual cusps
    c. a and b
    d. clearing wax mesially from contact areas for maxillary supporting cusps, and distally for mandibular supporting cusp contacts on maxillary teeth
    e. a, b, and d

Unit 6

Occlusal Examination and Articulation of Casts

In order to mount casts on an articulator effectively, certain kinds of data should be obtained and recorded at the time of the oral examination. Such information includes: (1) initial premature contact(s) in centric relation, (2) absence of centric stops, (3) mobile teeth, (4) working side contacts, (5) balancing side contacts, (6) protrusive contacts, and (7) facets of wear. This information is specifically related to mounting of the casts and is only a small part of that obtained in the comprehensive oral and occlusal examination. The examination is done before the casts are mounted to avoid an additional appointment to see if the casts are properly mounted.

INTRODUCTION: UNIT OBJECTIVES AND READING

The objective of this unit is to indicate the information that should be obtained in the oral examination in order to facilitate the correct mounting of casts in an articulator. Several behavorial objectives are considered.
A. Objectives
   1. Be able to list the information needed to effectively evaluate mounted casts when the patient is not available.
   2. Be able to indicate why information about occlusal contacts is needed.
   3. Be able to indicate the limitations of the application of the information to the articulation of the casts.
B. Reading (optional)
   Kerr, D. A., Ash, M. M., Jr., and Millaud, H. D.: Oral Diagnosis, 5th edition. St. Louis, C. V. Mosby Co., 1978 (Chapter 10).

EXAMINATION INFORMATION

The information can be obtained in any reasonable sequence. The best procedure is to verify the mounting when the patient is present; however, in most instances completion of the mounting occurs when the patient is not present.

Premature Contacts in Centric Relation

The location of the initial contact in centric relation must be the same on the articulated casts as in the patient. If it is not the same, the mandibular cast must be remounted correctly in centric relation.

A premature contact is an interference to

91

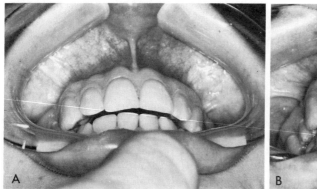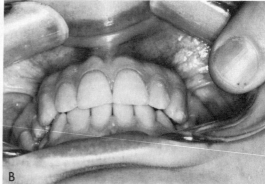

Figure 6–1. Occlusal interference. *A*, premature contact in centric relation; *B*, centric occlusion. A to B, slide in centric.

jaw closure into a stable intercuspal position (Fig. 6–1). It may be related to a lateral as well as an anterior slide into centric occlusion.

Centric Stops

The presence and absence of centric stops in the patient can be determined with articulating paper and shim stock.* Most of the stops present in the mouth should be present on the mounted casts when the casts are properly positioned in centric occlusion. The absence of major centric stops is usually due to an error in the centric relation check bite but may be due to the difference in the passive state of the teeth when an impression is taken and the active state of compression in centric

---

*Artus Corporation, Englewood, NJ 07631.

occlusion (as previously discussed under centric occlusion, Unit 1). In the mouth and on casts centric stops are often seen as a bull's eye (Fig. 6–2) when marked with articulating paper. Shim stock is used to determine the presence or absence of contact between only two opposing teeth or cusps at one time.

Mobile Teeth

All teeth should be tested for mobility. It is important to indicate the type and degree of mobility — lateral, vertical, and so forth. Mobile teeth tend to be displaced under compression when biting in centric occlusion (maximum intercuspation) and in lateral movements. Because of such mobility the position of the teeth on the casts may be different from their position in the mouth, and the discrepancy can prevent proper articulation in centric oc-

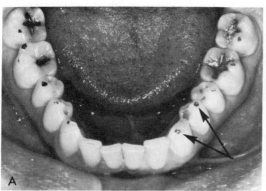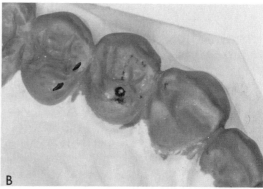

Figure 6–2. Centric stops. *A*, bull's eye centric stops on patient's teeth and *B*, on casts. Marks are due to flat surfaces (facets of wear).

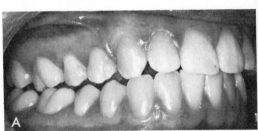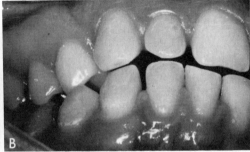

Figure 6–3. Working side contacts and interferences. A, working side contacts on cuspids and molars; B, disclusion of cuspids due to premature contacts on premolars.

clusion. The presence of mobile teeth, especially those that can be intruded, often involves a premature contact in centric occlusion. Tooth mobility should be evaluated by manual palpation statically and during movement of the jaw with the teeth in light contact. If a tooth can be intruded in the centric occlusion position, adjustment of that tooth on the cast may be necessary in order to obtain a proper mounting.

Working Side Contacts

Working side contacts that are present in the patient should be duplicated on the mounted casts (Fig. 6–3A). However, because of the limitations of an articulator all such contacts may not be possible. Multiple posterior contacts in lateral excursions (group function) are more difficult to duplicate on casts than single cuspid contacts (cuspid disclusion). If group function is to include posterior teeth, a suitable articulator must be used or compensatory pro-

cedures applied to obtain the function desired. For example, it is possible to obtain more contact during mounting of maxillary casts by elevating the plane of occlusion to be more parallel with the inclination of the condylar guidance in lateral excursions. Such procedures have limitations and should not be routinely practiced.

Working side interferences are contacts that interfere with smooth gliding movements, cause displacement or heavy contact on individual teeth, or cause disclusion when working side contacts should be present (Fig. 6–3B).

Balancing Side Contacts

The presence or absence of balancing side contacts in a patient has a direct relationship to setting the condylar guidance on the articulator (Fig. 6–4A). Considering some amount of discrepancy between centric relation and centric occlusion, the less the inclination of the condylar guidance of the articulator, the

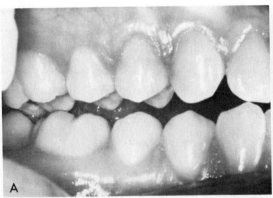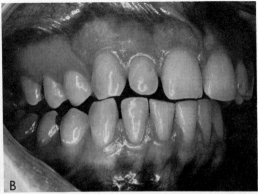

Figure 6–4. Balancing side contacts and interferences. A, right balancing side contact; B, disclusion on working side due to premature contact on left balancing side.

more likely there will be balancing side contacts in the lateral protrusive position, provided that contact has not been lost on the working side by decreasing the condylar inclination too far. For complete tooth guidance in waxing restorations, it is possible to decrease the condylar inclination to make certain that balancing contacts are made and balancing interferences avoided. In effect, the condylar inclination is reduced to maximize tooth guidance.

Balancing side interferences are contacts on the balancing side that cause disclusion of the teeth on the working side or displacement of teeth on the balancing side (Fig. 6–4B).

Protrusive Contacts

Any posterior contact during protrusive movements is considered to be undesirable. All guidance should be on anterior teeth and edge-to-edge contact of incisors should be possible (Fig. 6–5A). The amount of posterior contact on the casts on the articulator will depend upon the inclination of the condylar and incisal guidances of the articulator. Immediate disclusion occurs with steep inclinations of these guidances. However, in order for the clinician to wax restorations on articulated working casts while emphasizing tooth guidance, the guidance of the teeth should determine the inclination of these guidances. Thus the guidance should be set to maximize contact of the teeth when waxing restorations in order to avoid interferences in the restorations.

A *protrusive interference* is any interference to smooth gliding protrusive movements. Such an interference may cause anterior disclusion (Fig. 6–5B) or displacement of teeth as well as interfere with a straight forward movement with the teeth in contact.

Facets of Wear

Facets of wear may be caused by function and parafunction (bruxism). Patterns of wear may relate to ongoing activity or to past bruxism. If contacts can be made between facets of wear in the patient (Fig. 6–6), it should be possible to make such contacts on the articulated casts. In some instances it may not be possible for the patient to cause facets of wear to make contact because the occlusion has changed. Such changes may have resulted from orthodontics, restorations, temporomandibular joint–muscle dysfunction, periodontal disease, bruxism, caries, or trauma (accidents, fractures, and so forth). In some instances of temporomandibular joint dysfunction contact may be present one day and absent the next.

If facets of wear do not make contact on the articulated casts, the mandibular cast may not be mounted correctly in centric relation. And if the casts cannot be articulated fully in centric occlusion, it will not be possible to have facets of wear make contact in lateral movements. In order to differentiate between the absence of occlusal contact relations in the mouth and an absence of contacts on the articulated casts, it is necessary to know if the contacts are present in the mouth, and where they are present.

Testing of occlusal contacts should be

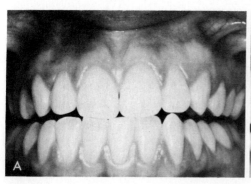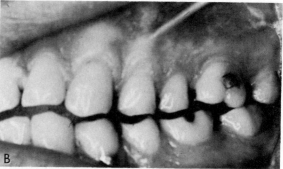

Figure 6–5. Protrusive contacts and interferences. *A,* edge-to-edge protrusive contacts; *B,* premature contact on second molar preventing anterior contact in lateral protrusive movement.

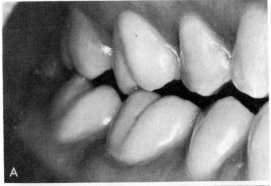
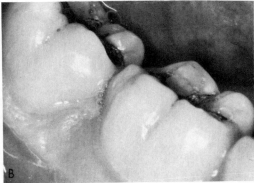
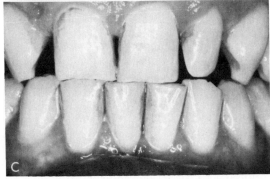

Figure 6–6. Facets of wear. *A,* working side contacts; *B,* facets of wear (same teeth as shown in A); *C,* anterior bruxing facets of wear.

made with shim stock with the incisal pin raised (or the incisal guidance customized) and the condylar guidances unlocked and free to be moved to obtain the best contacts. The evaluation of contacts on casts and in the mouth should be made with shim stock having the same thickness (.0005 in).

If contacts cannot be made between facets of wear in excursive movements, and the disclusion is not caused by an interference, and the articulator being used cannot be adjusted further, some consideration may be given to using another articulator for that case or to using compensating techniques involving adjustment of the maxillary cast with shims during certain movements. Some articulators allow for customizing of the condylar as

well as incisal guidance, and others allow for up-and-down adjustment of the position of the condylar elements. However, complete duplication of contacts is seldom possible using any articulator, and some compensation in waxing is often necessary. Such compensation will decrease the amount of adjustment (grinding) of the restorations when placed in the mouth.

When restorations are placed in the mouth, they should not interfere with contacts between facets of wear. Guidance by the clinician to the functional and parafunctional facets of wear is usually necessary. Occlusal interferences usually cause resistance to guidance, and avoidance to interferences, as reflected by muscle resistance, helps signal the presence of interferences to the clinicians.

Unit 6 Exercises

1. What information should be obtained from the oral examination in order to facilitate mounting of casts on an articulator?

   _____

2. Why is information about intraoral occlusal contact relations of value in mounting casts on an articulator?

   _____

   _____

3. What are the limitations on the use of the data obtained during the examination relative to mounting of casts on an articulator?

   _____

4. What is the effect of mobile teeth on an accurate mounting of casts on an articulator?

   _____

5. What is an interference called that involves the buccal slope of the lingual cusp of the lower first molar and the axial surface of the lingual cusp of the maxillary first molar?

   _____

6. Do centric stops remain the same for long periods of time in most instances? (yes, no). Under what conditions may they change?

   _____

7. A single cusp in contact on the working side can be considered an occlusal

   interference if_____

   _____.

8. The reason(s) that a patient cannot make facets of wear contact in the mouth include:

   _____

   _____

9. The reason(s) that facets of wear cannot be made to contact on mounted casts include:

   _____

   _____

10. What may be the significance of facets of wear not making contact in the mouth and on articulated casts?

_____

_____

Unit 6 Test

1. What is the significance of the absence of centric stops in the mouth?

   a. possible temporomandibular joint dysfunction
   b. shifting of teeth has occurred
   c. some restorations "too high"
   d. excessive occlusal adjustment
   e. all of the above

2. If centric stops are present in the mouth but absent on articulated casts:

   a. the mounting is probably incorrect
   b. the cast may be distorted
   c. a and b
   d. the teeth have shifted
   e. a, b, and d

3. A balancing side interference results in working side disclusion. This information is necessary:

   a. for setting the condylar inclination
   b. for taking a protrusive check bite
   c. for setting the lateral wings of the incisal table
   d. for setting the incisal guide inclination
   e. all of the above

4. A balancing side interference is found on articulated casts but not in the patient. This discrepancy is possibly because:

   a. the condylar inclination is incorrect
   b. the balancing interference tooth is mobile
   c. working side disclusion is not found when in fact it is present in the patient
   d. there is distortion of impression and hence distorted casts
   e. all of the above

5. The point of contact on a tooth when the jaw is guided into centric relation contact:

   a. cannot be used as a guide to proper mounting of casts
   b. cannot be duplicated precisely ($\pm$ 0.5 mm)
   c. a and b
   d. is used to evaluate mounting of casts
   e. a, b, and d

6. If the condylar inclination is changed to provide balancing side contacts (not interferences) to prevent balancing interference in waxing a restoration:

    a. it may not be possible to have centric stops in centric occlusion if the condylar inclination is not adjusted for the centric occlusion position
    b. there should be no disclusion on the working side
    c. no adjustment of the inclination for centric relation position is necessary
    d. the condylar inclination should be adjusted for the centric occlusion position
    e. all of the above

7. It is not possible to mount a set of casts correctly in centric relation and be able to position them in centric occlusion if:

    a. a tooth is in supraversion except when the patient bites into centric occlusion
    b. the molar teeth are quite mobile
    c. a and b
    d. the wax for centric relation registration bite is not thoroughly heat softened
    e. a, b, and d

8. If a patient is highly resistant to jaw movement in centric relation:

    a. mounting of casts correctly may be impossible at that time
    b. molar centric stops on mounted casts are likely to be absent using thin shim stock
    c. a and b
    d. the casts should be mounted in centric occlusion
    e. a, b, and d

9. If facets of wear make contact on mounted casts and are not present in the patient:

    a. casts were made prior to a change in the occlusion
    b. occlusion may have shifted after casts were made
    c. a and b
    d. distortion of impressions and casts may have taken place
    e. a, b, and d

10. Between the times that impressions have been taken (casts made) and the mounting of the casts, a patient has third molars extracted. The occlusal contacts on the casts do not match those in the mouth. The reason for the discrepancy is:

    a. change in temporomandibular joints
    b. change in occlusion
    c. a and b
    d. change in muscles
    e. a, b, and d

Unit 7

Mounting of Casts

Some of the principles for mounting casts on an articulator have been discussed in the preceding units. The primary objective of this unit is to present the procedures for mounting casts on a semi-adjustable articulator using a simple face bow, a centric relation registration, and a protrusive check bite. Both the use of the simple face bow (the non ear piece and the ear piece types) and the hinge axis locator will be discussed, but the latter only briefly for purposes of orientation. Simulation methods for mounting maxillary and mandibular casts have been included here to facilitate study of the mounting procedures in the laboratory.

INTRODUCTION: UNIT OBJECTIVES AND READING

The procedures for mounting casts include taking impressions to make casts to be articulated; however, this important procedure will be presented in outline form only. The importance of examination of the patient's occlusion as it relates to mounting of casts has already been discussed in Unit 6.

A. Objectives
   1. Be able to describe:
      a. procedures for mounting the maxillary cast using the (1) non ear piece face bow, and (2) the ear piece face bow.
      b. procedures for mounting the mandibular cast in centric relation.
   2. Be able to describe and carry out procedures for mounting maxillary and mandibular casts using simulation methods.
   3. Be able to describe and carry out procedures for setting the horizontal

and lateral condylar guidance inclinations on the Hanau H2 articulator.

B. Reading (optional)
   Ramfjord, S. P., and Ash, M. M., Jr.: Occlusion. Philadelphia, W. B. Saunders Co., 1971 (Chapter 10).

IMPRESSIONS AND CASTS

A number of factors are responsible for obtaining good impressions, but only three will be briefly discussed inasmuch as most of the errors in making diagnostic casts arise because of (1) surface imperfections related to plaque and bubbles trapped on the teeth, (2) incorrect tray size, and (3) excessive pressure on the tray so that one or more cusp tips penetrate the impression material and make contact with the tray.

The first problem involves cleaning the teeth. The second problem can be avoided by simply checking the periphery of the

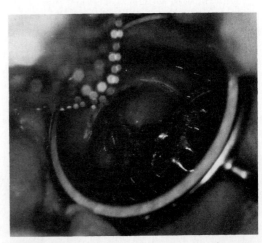

Figure 7-1. Impression tray not covering distal molar will result in inadequate casts.

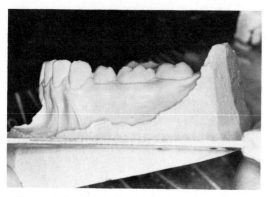

Figure 7–2. Base of cast should be trimmed parallel with the occlusal plane to facilitate mounting, especially with the splint cast technique.

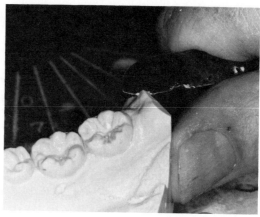

Figure 7–3. Retromolar areas may be an interference in balancing and working and should be trimmed.

tray with a mouth mirror (Fig. 7–1). The third problem is avoided by positioning the tray correctly and applying the correct amount of pressure.

Several problems may arise in pouring the stone into the impressions, but the principal error involves entrapment of air so that voids, or "peduncles," appear on the surface of the casts. Proper mixing of stone (in a vacuum) and use of a vibrator is the first step in avoiding this error. Pouring the stone into the impression requires that slight moisture be present on the surface of the impression and that a small amount of stone be vibrated along from tooth to tooth.

Trimming the base of diagnostic casts (Fig. 7–2) is somewhat cosmetic but in many respects very functional if a split cast method is used in making a splint. Nothing should prevent the occlusal surfaces from coming together in all areas. Possible contacts between stone rather than teeth that may prevent occlusal contact in lateral positions and excursion should be removed (Fig. 7–3).

QUICK LOOK AT MOUNTING PROCEDURES

A brief outline of the steps in the face bow transfer and mounting of casts is given in Figure 7–4. For nonclinical appli-cations refer to the section on simulation methods of mounting casts, p. 113.

Steps in Mounting Casts

Step 1. *Face Bow Registration*

a. Place the wax on the bite plane (or bite fork) and press into position on maxillary teeth (Fig. 7–4A).

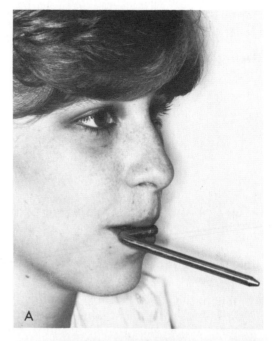

b. Remove the bite plane and chill wax. Impressions of the cusps should be present (Fig. 7–4B). Chill and return to the mouth.

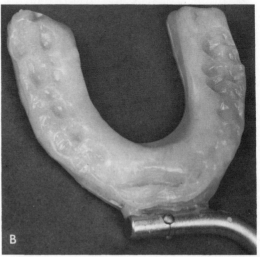

c. Place the face bow on the bite plane and center ear piece or non ear piece face bow on the head. Lock in position.

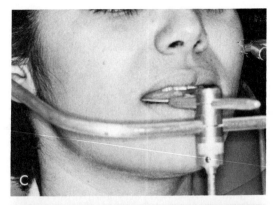

Step 2. *Face Bow Transfer*

a. Center the face bow on the articular and attach the maxillary cast to the upper member with plaster (Fig. 7–4D).

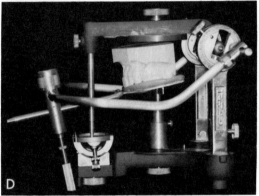

Step 3. *Centric Relation Registration*

a. Obtain a centric relation check bite record to relate the mandibular cast to the hinge axis of the articulator and to the maxillary cast (Fig. 7–4E).

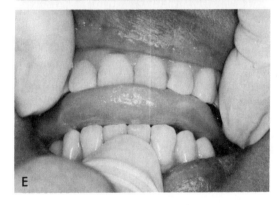

Step 4. *Mounting of Mandibular Cast*

a. Using the wax check bite mount the mandibular cast using a mounting stand (Fig. 7–4F).

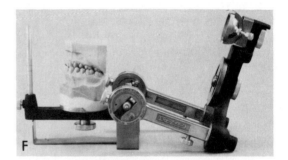

Step 5. *"Functional" Records*

a. Complete mounting with setting of horizontal and lateral condylar inclinations (Fig. 7–4G) with protrusive check bite.

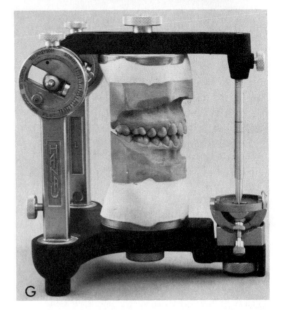

RELATING THE MAXILLA TO THE PATIENT'S HINGE AXIS

The first step in mounting the maxillary cast is relating the maxilla to the patient's hinge axis with a face bow. This step will be limited to use of an arbitrary hinge axis rather than the "true" hinge axis. The potential error from using the arbitrary axis is discussed in Unit 8. The Hanau non ear piece and ear piece face bow will be discussed.

FACE BOW REGISTRATION

The relationship of the maxillary arch to the hinge axis is registered with a face bow (kinematic or simple). The kinematic face bow or hinge axis locator establishes the terminal or "true" hinge axis; the simple face bow relates the maxillary arch to an "arbitrary" hinge axis. A brief review of the method of locating the terminal hinge axis is given as a basis of orientation. Although not commonly used now, an estimate (measurement) of the hinge axis is helpful for understanding the "automatic" method of obtaining the hinge axis.

Locating the Terminal Hinge Axis

The terminal hinge axis is found with a kinematic face bow or a hinge axis locator. The principle for locating the hinge axis rests on rotary movement of the mandible without translation in centric relation.

Hinge Axis Locator

A hinge axis locator or a kinematic face bow makes use of clutches attached to the upper and lower arches and adjustable rods attached to the clutches (Fig. 7–5). At the end of each rod attached to the lower clutch is a stylus. The upper rod on each side has a flag and each lower rod is adjusted to position the stylus over a dot on the flag. When pure rotary motion is obtained (the stylus does not move off from a point), the mandible is indicated to be in centric relation (condyles in rearmost

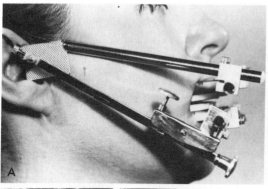
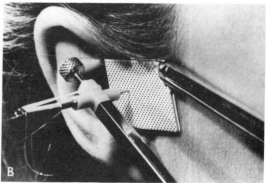
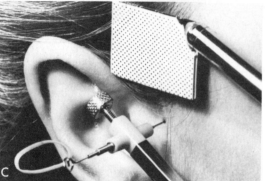

Figure 7–5. Locating terminal hinge axis. Use of hinge axis locator. *A,* clutches on both arches with adjustable rods for stylus (lower) and flag (upper); *B,* stylus in position of only rotary movement; *C,* flag up and stylus in position to mark terminal hinge axis.

uppermost position) and the axis of rotation is the true hinge axis. In the absence of functional disturbances this axis is quite reproducible (± 0.5 mm).

Locating the Arbitrary Hinge Axis

There are minor variations in the steps for locating the hinge axis, depending on the type of face bow and articulator being used. The two common methods of locating the arbitrary hinge axis are the measurement method using the non ear piece face bow and the automatic method using the ear piece face bow. The different methods are related to the type of face bow used. Non ear piece face bow (Hanau) is related to the measured (arbitrary) hinge axis (Fig. 7–6A) and supported on the condylar shaft of the articulator (Fig. 7–6B). Ear piece face bow (Hanau) automatically locates arbitrary hinge axis and is supported on the articular by pins located on the centric locks (Fig. 7–6B).

Measurement Method of Locating Arbitrary Hinge Axis (Non Ear Piece Method)

1. Place a flexible rule on a line from the posterior border of the middle of the tragus of the ear to the outer canthus of the eye (Fig. 7–7A).
2. With a felt tip pen or ballpoint pen, place a mark 12 to 13 mm anterior to the border of the tragus. This marks the point of the arbitrary hinge axis (Fig. 7–7B).

Preparing the Bite Plane (Ear Piece and Non Ear Piece Methods)

Before using the simple face bow to register the relationship for transfer to the articulator, the bite plane must be prepared as follows:
1. Place several thicknesses of wax on a heated plane or bite fork and seal to the metal (Fig. 7–8).
2. Soften the wax on the bite fork with a

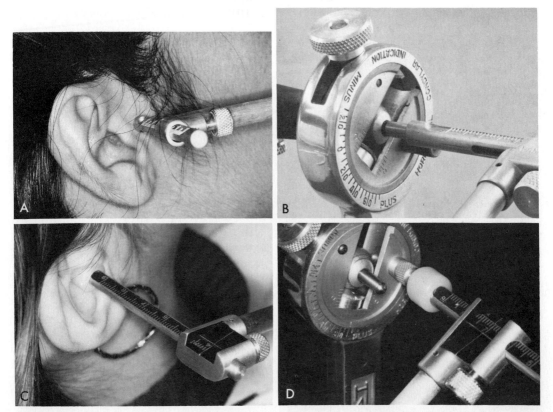

Figure 7–6. Use of face bow. *A*, non ear piece face bow related to arbitrary hinge axis and *B*, supported on axis shaft of the articulator. *C*, ear piece face bow in position to locate hinge axis; and *D*, supported on centric lock pin.

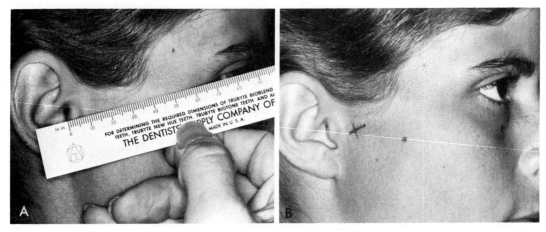

Figure 7–7. Locating arbitrary hinge axis. *A*, measurement of hinge axis; *B*, mark locating arbitrary hinge axis.

flame, temper it in a bowl of hot water or a hot water bath, and push the bite fork with wax onto the maxillary teeth to make indentations as shown in Figure 7–9*A*,*B*.

3. Remove the bite fork, chill in cold water and remove excess wax with a sharp knife. The cusp tips should not penetrate the wax to the metal bite fork and should be free of soft tissue impingement. If the metal has been touched, redo steps 1 and 2. It is not necessary to obtain very deep penetration of cusp tips or to obtain an impression of every single cusp tip. There should be sufficient indentation of anterior and posterior teeth to have a good stable base for the cast and to be certain of the occlusal plane.

4. Replace the bite fork in the mouth. The patient can hold the bite fork in position when cotton rolls are placed under it. The patient is instructed to close his or her jaw slowly but firmly and slightly forward (protrusive) against the cotton rolls (Fig. 7–10).

5. When the bite fork is stable, insert the bite fork stem into the bite fork clamp of the face bow.

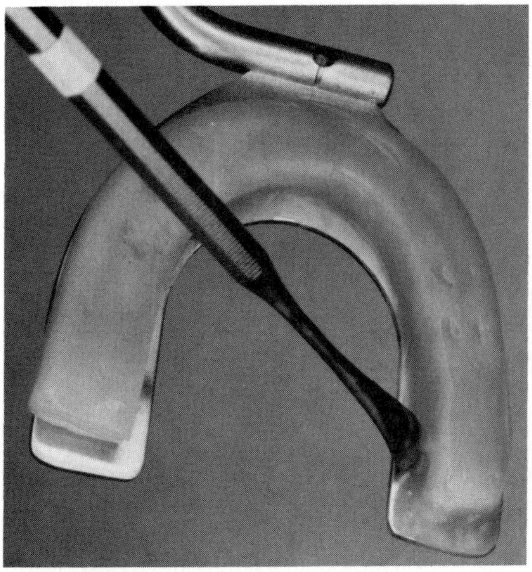

Non Ear Piece Face Bow Registration

1. Adjust the bite plane stem on the bite clamp, place each hinge axis rod over the arbitrary hinge axis points that were measured on the patient, and center the face bow. After centering the face bow, lock the bite clamp and check the position of the axis rods over the hinge axis points (Fig. 7–11). The axis rods of the face bow should just touch the skin over the arbitrary hinge axis points.

2. If your face bow and articulator are not equipped with an infraorbital pointer, skip to 3. If the infraorbital pointer is present, set the pointer to the infraorbital notch (Fig. 7–12). The infraorbital pointer is used to establish the third point of reference for the face bow (see Figure 4–4).

3. When the face bow has been centered on the patient, remove the face bow and transfer to articulator.

Figure 7–8. Preparation of bite plane. Several thicknesses of wax sealed to bite plane.

Figure 7–9. Preparation of bite plane. *A,* bite plane with warmed wax is positioned on maxillary teeth and wax chilled; *B,* prepared bite plane.

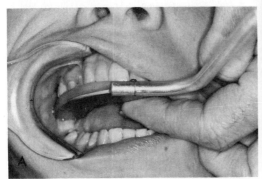

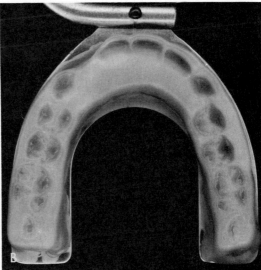

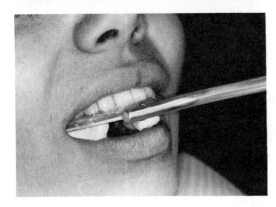

Figure 7–10. Stabilization of bite plane. Use of cotton rolls to hold bite plane in position.

Figure 7–11. Face bow registration. Registration if relationship of maxillary arch to the measured hinge axis is completed after centering and locking the face bow.

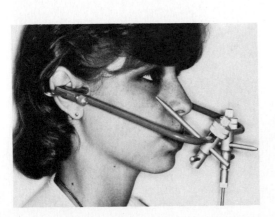

Figure 7–12. Face bow registration. Infraorbital notch can be determined on the patient and used for the third point of reference on the articulator.

4. Proceed to p. 109 for *Relating Maxillary Arch (Cast) to the Articulator Hinge Axis* (Face Bow Transfer).

Ear Piece Face Bow Registration

1. After the bite fork has been prepared and inserted into the patient's mouth, its stem or handle is to be inserted into the bite fork clamp of the face bow.

2. Slightly unturn the two frame thumbscrews and slide the scales outward to maximize the opening between the nylon ear pieces (Fig. 7–13). The nylon ear pieces are threaded onto the scales and may be removed for cold sterilization.

3. The face bow is then brought gently over the face with the stem of the bite plane or bite fork entering the opened clamp.

4. Hold both frame thumbscrews between the thumbs and middle fingers. Place forefingers on the ends of the scales and slide them to enter the nylon ear pieces into the meatus of the ear (Fig. 7–14A).

5. Simultaneously slide the frames laterally to symmetrically adjust the scales while maintaining a comfortable yet secure suspension of the nylon ear pieces in the meatus. Tighten both frame thumbscrews to maintain this symmetry of suspension.

6. Grasp the frontal portion of the face bow and tighten the clamp thumbscrew securely to lock this relationship of bow to

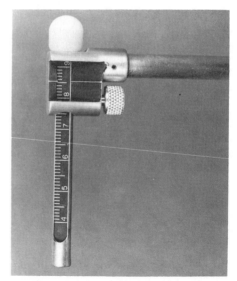

Figure 7–13. Ear piece face bow. Set the ear piece on one side to minimum and the other side to maximum. Place ear piece of maximum side into ear and move minimum side into ear in position. Add the two sides together and divide by two to determine proper separation of ear pieces.

bite plane or bite fork (Fig. 7–14B). Do not distort the position of the face bow frame during tightening of the thumbscrew.

7. Release the two frame thumbscrews and withdraw the scales with nylon ear pieces from the meatus.

8. Remove the entire face bow assembly from the patient's mouth.

9. See the following discussion for face bow transfer.

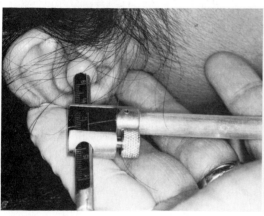
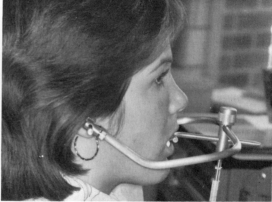

Figure 7–14. Ear piece face bow registration. *A*, position nylon ear pieces in ear as indicated; *B*, securely lock face bow in position to complete registration.

RELATING THE MAXILLARY ARCH (CAST) TO THE ARTICULAR HINGE AXIS (FACE BOW TRANSFER)

The procedures for the simple non ear piece face bow and ear piece face bow differ in that the ear piece is placed in a different position on the Hanau H2–PR from where it is on the simple face bow. On the non ear piece face bow the axis rods of the face bow are centered on the ends of the condylar shafts; on the ear rod face bow the face bow is centered on the pin projecting from the centric lock. Note also the measurement from the pin to the condylar shaft and relate this to the measurement of the distance from the tragus to the hinge axis points (Fig. 7–15). The phrase "face bow transfer" refers to the transfer of the relationship between the maxillary arch and the hinge axis to an articulator.

Non Ear Piece Face Bow Transfer

1. Set horizontal condylar guidances of the articulator to 0° and the lateral guidance to 0°.
2. Lock the condylar elements against the centric stops. The articulator must be at "zero" centric.
3. Center the face bow condylar rods on the articulator shafts (Fig. 7–16). The average for center on this type of face bow is 6.5. However, because they get bent sometimes, face bows must be centered individually.

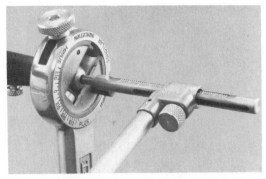

Figure 7–16. Non ear piece face bow transfer. Face bow condylar rods are supported on the axis shaft of the articulator.

4. The anterior (third point) of reference is between the middle notches on the incisal pin. The face bow is raised until the incisal edges of the maxillary teeth are at the same height as the notch.
5. Proceed to p. 110 for mounting maxillary cast to complete transfer.

Ear Piece Face Bow Transfer

1. Check the articulator to make sure it is in zero centric.
2. Set the condylar inclination to 70° (Fig. 7–17); the degree lateral inclination should be zero.

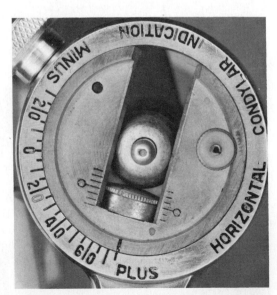

Figure 7–17. Ear piece face bow transfer. With the ear piece face bow the condylar inclination *must* be set to 70 degrees to automatically relate to the hinge axis.

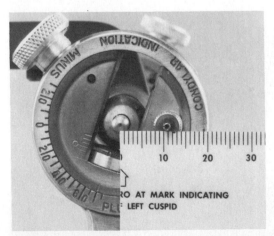

Figure 7–15. Ear piece face bow transfer. When condylar inclination is set to 70 degrees the ear piece is set 11 to 12 mm from the hinge axis of the articulator.

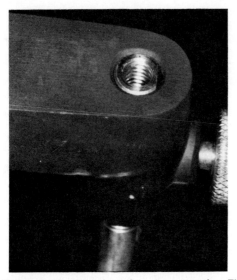

Figure 7–18. Ear piece face bow transfer. The articulator must be set at zero. Unless the pin is flush with the top surface, the pin will not contact the incisal table at its center.

3. Centric locks are tightened to restrict the articulator to opening and closing movements only.

4. Make certain the incisal pin is flush with the articulator's top surface (Fig. 7–18).

5. Roughen the surface of the base of the cast with a knife for retention or key for split cast mounting (Fig. 7–19).

6. Attach the mounting ring to the upper member. Make sure the pin is located in the slot at the base of the ring (Fig. 7–20).

7. Soak the base of the cast in water for retention, or use separating medium for split cast mounting.

8. Attach the ear pieces of the face bow assembly to the pin on each condylar lock (Fig. 7–21) and adjust the movable rods for equal numbers on each side.

9. With the adjustable screw on the bottom of the bite fork support clamp, raise or lower the bite plane until it reaches the level of the lower notch on the incisal pin. For the ear piece face bow, the incisal edges of the central incisors should be 58 mm above the level of the surface of the lower member of the articulator.

10. Proceed to next discussion to complete transfer.

Mounting Maxillary Cast

1. Seat the maxillary cast into the indentations in the wax on the bite fork (Fig. 7–22). Support the cast with a telescoping

Figure 7–19. Face bow transfer. Cast must be roughened to provide retention unless a split cast mount is to be done.

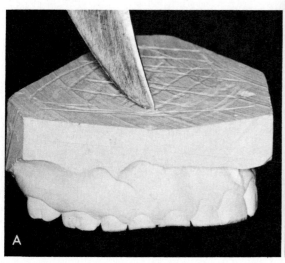

A

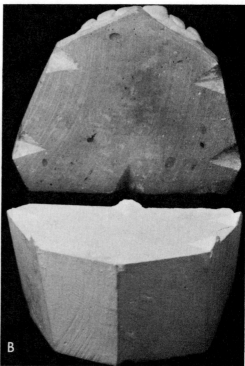

B

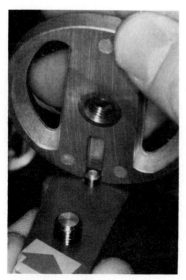

Figure 7–20. Attachment of mounting ring. Orientation pin must lie in slot on mounting ring to be able to remove and replace cast in the same position.

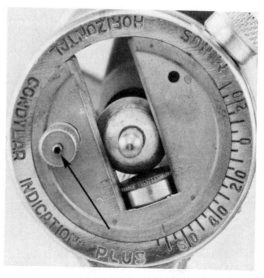

Figure 7–21. Ear piece face bow transfer. The face bow is supported by the pin indicated by arrow to the condylar lock.

support. Attach the cast to the mounting ring with a creamy mixture of impression plaster.

RELATING THE MANDIBLE (CAST) TO CENTRIC RELATION, TO THE MAXILLARY (CAST), AND TO THE HINGE AXIS OF THE ARTICULATOR

Centric relation and centric occlusion are probably the two most commonly used maxillomandibular positions. These positions may be recorded with a variety of materials including wax, but only the use of wax will be described here. Restorations completed with casts malaligned in their starting position will have premature contacts and occlusal interferences when inserted in the mouth.

Centric Relation Check Bite

1. Train the patient in relaxation in order to guide the mandible into centric relation.

2. Prepare two to three layers of pink

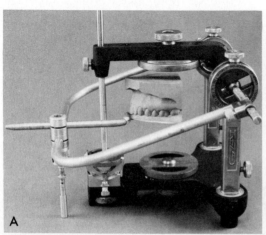

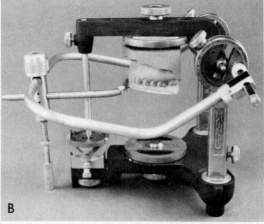

Figure 7–22. Face bow transfer. Mounting of maxillary cast. Cast is positioned with condylar rods set: *A,* on axle of articulator for non ear piece face bow; or *B,* on condylar lock pin for the ear piece face bow.

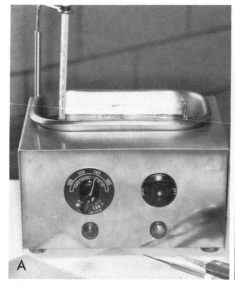
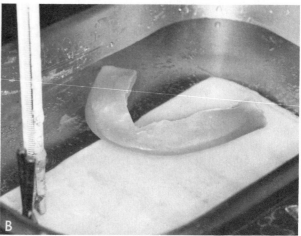

Figure 7–23. Centric relation check bite. *A, B,* centric relation registration for the mounting of the mandibular cast uses a wax rim heated in a water bath.

base plate wax in the shape and length of the maxillary arch. Place in a water bath with temperature of 138° F (Fig. 7–23A,B).

3. Place softened wax on the teeth of the maxillary arch and guide the mandible into the wax. Do not allow the teeth to make contact or let the patient bite into the wax. The wax must be soft and the teeth guided by the operator into the wax.

4. Trim away excess wax (Fig. 7–24A).

5. Chill the wax (Fig. 7–24B).

6. Trim excess wax from the surface of the wax check bite.

7. In the clinical situation a protrusive registration at this time is indicated. However, the procedure is presented on p. 115,

under *Functional Records for Setting the H2–PR Articulator.*

Mounting Mandibular Cast in Centric Relation

1. Relate the mandibular cast to the maxillary cast with the check bite. Do not force casts into wax. Trim wax to allow the casts to sit easily in the check bite.

2. Drop pin 2 to 3 mm to account for check bite thickness (Fig. 7–25). Set the horizontal condylar inclination at 25.

3. With the articulator inverted on the mounting stand (Fig. 7–26A), hold the mandibular and the maxillary cast together

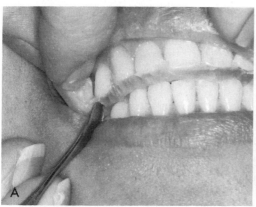
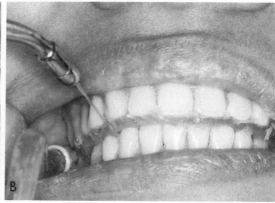

Figure 7–24. Centric relation registration. *A,* wax is trimmed to allow proper seating of the cast; *B,* wax is cooled before removal from teeth.

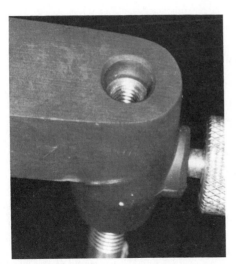

Figure 7–25. Mounting mandibular cast. Drop the pin a distance equal to the thickness of the wax so that the incisal pin (off-set) can be adjusted to the center of the incisal table.

in the CR check bite relationship. Attach with a creamy mixture of impression plaster. After plaster has set remove check bite.

4. Raise the incisal pin. Close the casts into centric occlusion and drop the pin to contact on the incisal table (Fig. 7–26 B).

5. Proceed to p. 116 for setting the horizontal and lateral condylar inclination.

SIMULATION METHODS FOR FACE BOW TRANSFER AND MOUNTING OF CASTS

Simulated Face Bow Transfer

For laboratory exercises the face bow may be used to position and support the maxillary cast. Two general principles related to the concept of waxing restorations to maximize tooth guidance are followed to the extent possible: (1) place the maxillary cast forward (but allow for clearance of incisal table) and center cast laterally, (2) make the occlusal plane as parallel as possible with a low inclination of the condylar guidance (10° to 15°) and raised as high as possible without the cast hitting the mounting ring. The occlusal plane should not be inclined upward posteriorly more than 15°. The general principle is to reduce as much as possible the control of the condylar guidance of the articulator over the casts, i.e., increase tooth guidance, reduce articulator condylar guidance.

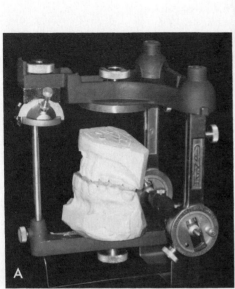
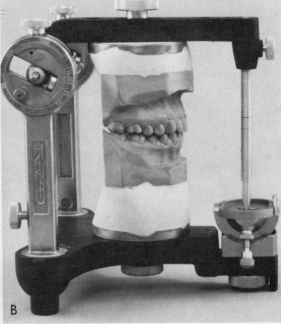

Figure 7–26. Mounting mandibular cast in centric relation. *A*, cast is seated securely in the wax check bite and held by hand while being attached to mounting ring with quick setting impression plaster; *B*, incisal pin set in contact with table with casts in centric occlusion. If it cannot be centered using the straight pin, the off-set pin is used.

Mounting of Mandibular Cast in Simulated Centric Relation (For Slide in Centric)

The mandibular cast may be mounted in a simulated centric occlusion for study purposes and for waxing a splint for a patient with muscle hypertonicity or temporomandibular joint dysfunction. A simulated centric relation mounting of the mandibular cast is used also as a teaching device in the laboratory and in selected instances of restorative treatment when a good CR check bite is impossible to obtain, viz., in temporomandibular joint–muscle pain dysfunction. In order to simulate a centric relation mounting on the Hanau H2–PR, the PR adjustment is used as in 1a and 2a. If a Hanau H2–PR articulator is not being used, follow steps 1b and 2b.

1a. Unlock the condylar stop locks and move the centric stops counterclockwise for 1 mm and reset the locks (Fig. 7–27A). If a lateral slide in centric is desired, set one side clockwise 1 mm and the other side ½ or ¾ mm counterclockwise.

b. Insert a metal or plastic shim (1 mm thick) between the condylar stop and condylar element) (Fig. 7–27B).

2a. Keeping the condylar element in contact with the condylar stop, reset the condylar lock.

b. Keeping the condylar element in contact with the shim, reset the condylar lock.

3. Position the mandibular cast into maxillary cast in centric occlusion (maximum interdigitation).

4. With the articulator inverted in the mounted stand, hold the mandibular cast in centric occlusion and attach to the lower member of the articulator with a creamy mixture of impression plaster.

5. After the plaster sets, reset the condylar stop back to zero. When the condylar elements are forward, in contact with the condylar stops, the cast-to-cast relation is centric relation. When the casts are in maximum interdigitation (centric occlusion), the condylar elements are in centric occlusion and the discrepancy between centric relation and centric occlusion is 1 mm.

Simulated Mounting of Maxillary Cast for Centric Relation (Clinical Convenience)

When it is apparent that a centric relation check bite is inadequate because the

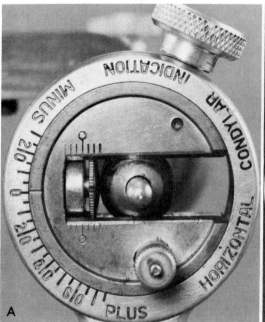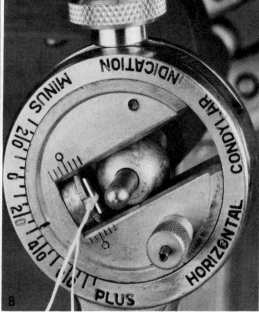

Figure 7–27. Mounting mandibular cast in simulated centric relation. *A,* centric stop moved clockwise 1 mm to produce a one millimeter slide in centric; *B,* use of shim to accomplish same result as in *A.* The condylar element in both *A* and *B* is in the centric occlusion position.

casts do not occlude in centric occlusion (absent posterior stops), but the slide in centric and the premature contact in centric relation are acceptable, the maxillary cast can be remounted to obtain a reasonable mounting for centric relation. Such a mounting can be used for study purposes and for some restorative procedures. It is a clinical convenience in that another centric check bite is not required and the method is used principally for expediency.

Step 1. Set condylar guidance with protrusive check bite or by method described on p. 118.

Step 2. Loosen the condylar guide locks and the thumbnut for the mounting ring of the maxillary cast. Position the maxillary cast in centric occlusion.

Step 3. Rotate the condylar stop counterclockwise until it just makes light contact with the condylar element. Lock the centric stops and the condylar guide locks.

Step 4. Remove the maxillary cast from the articulator and separate the cast from the mounting ring at the mounting ring. With a model trimmer, reduce the plaster to provide space for the mounting ring. Replace the mounting ring on the articulator. The incisal pin is centered and flush with the upper surface of the articulator's upper member.

Step 5. Place the maxillary cast in centric occlusion on the mandibular cast (which is still mounted on the articulator). While holding the casts firmly in position in centric occlusion, mount the maxillary cast to the mounting ring with impression plaster.

Step 6. Unlock the centric stop locks and rotate clockwise unitl at zero position. Unlock the condylar guide locks.

Step 7. Check for all contact relations of casts: centric occlusion, centric relation, working, balancing, and protrusive positions.

All occlusal contacts should reasonably approximate those of the patient as indicated in the patient's examination record, and the vertical, horizontal (anteroposterior), and lateral components of the slide in centric should closely approximate those in the patient. If they do not, the casts will have to be remounted with new check bites.

FUNCTIONAL RECORDS FOR SETTING THE H2–PR ARTICULATOR

The functional records for the Hanau H2 and H2–PR articulator and other articulators are not set by true functional records. Securing functional records refers to the registration of jaw positions (viz., centric relation and protrusive check bites) and approximations of the condylar paths using instruments such as the pantograph. Two inclinations are set from a protrusive registration: (1) condylar inclination and (2) lateral inclination. The latter is computed by formula, as indicated earlier.

Obtaining the Protrusive Record

As in obtaining any registration record, it is necessary to train the patient in the movements expected of him or her, and to go through the procedure as required to obtain the correct check bite. Have the wax record thoroughly heated before attempting the registration.

1. Fabricate the wax bite to be three to

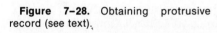

Figure 7–28. Obtaining protrusive record (see text).

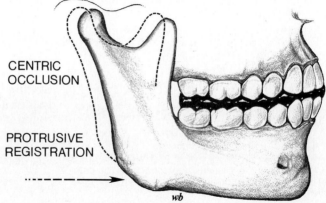

CENTRIC OCCLUSION

PROTRUSIVE REGISTRATION

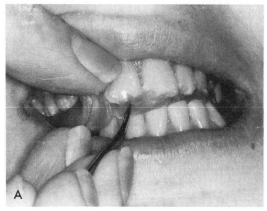 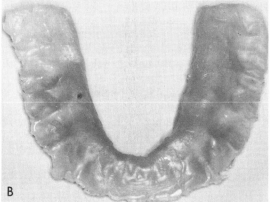

Figure 7–29. Obtaining protrusive record. *A, B,* trim wax to allow proper registration of casts.

four layers thick in the posterior and two layers thick in the anterior part of the mouth.

2. When guiding the patient's mandible into protrusive contact with the softened wax, do not allow the patient to make edge-to-edge contact of the teeth. The anterior protrusion should not be more than 4 to 5 mm anterior to centric relation or centric occlusion (Fig. 7–28).

3. Guide the patient into a straight protrusive position several times and check the position of the midlines of the arches to see if you have guided the patient straight forward from centric relation. With the wax bite heated thoroughly and held against the maxillary dentition, instruct the patient to close into the protrusive relation short of tooth contact. Do not allow the patient to bite through the wax. Check to see if the midlines are in the same position as in centric relation.

4. Trim wax away from buccal surfaces of the teeth with a small wax spatula (Fig. 7–29A).

5. Chill the wax and trim superior and inferior surfaces in order to avoid soft tissue impingements and to allow accurate cast positioning (Fig. 7–29B).

In Figure 7–30 the path of the condyle is curved (CP), but the condylar guidance path of the articulator is straight (SP). If the path is viewed from CR to P and the condylar guidance (CG) is set on the basis of a shorter protrusive (P_1) check bite rather than the longer P, the problem of a curved versus straight condylar guidance will be minimized. Since an increase in condylar guidance results in a raising of the maxillary cast, the maintenance of centric stop contacts must be tested in relation to the condylar guidance. The protrusive check bite must be minimal (no more or less than 4 to 5 mm), but sufficient to obtain an adequate record. In general, the greater the protrusion, the greater the chance for error. Actually, a protrusion of 4 to 5 mm is a compromise between the physiologically desirable (less than 4 mm) and the mechanically possible. This topic will be discussed in further detail in Unit 8.

Setting the Horizontal Condylar Inclination and Lateral Condylar Inclination

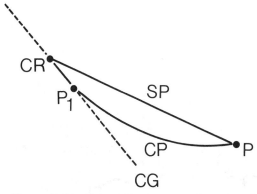

Figure 7–30. Schematic representation of path of condyle and relation to protrusive registration (see text).

(If a protrusive record is not available, proceed to *Setting of Horizontal Condylar Inclination Without Protrusive Check Bite,* p. 118.)

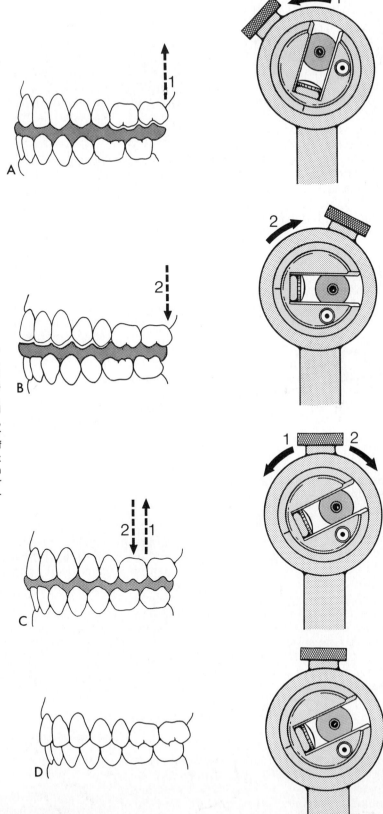

Figure 7–31. Setting horizontal condylar inclination. *A,* Condylar inclination increased (1) and back of maxillary cast is tipped up at molar area (1); *B,* condylar inclination decreased (2) and cast tipped down (2), causing opening in the anterior area; *C,* point of no tipping of cast (1) (2); *D,* protrusive wax check bite removed and casts in centric occlusion and condylar element in centric occlusion position.

1. Loosen the condylar guide thumb-nuts and centric locks to allow the upper member of the articulator to move freely.

2. Raise the upper member of the artic-ulator and place the protrusive wax rec-ord on the mandibular cast. Move the upper member of the articulator until the maxillary cast fits into the protrusive rec-ord.

3. Holding the upper and lower members of the articulator firmly together, move the horizontal condylar guidance thumbnut forward (1) as shown in Fig. 7–31A and backward (2) as shown in Fig. 7–31B until a position is found in which the maxillary cast does not rock in the protrusive check bite (Fig. 7–31C). Tight-en the condylar guidance thumbnut. Du-plicate on the opposite side and note the horizontal guidance inclinations. The dis-tance from the condylar element to the condylar stop should be nearly equal on both sides. The incisal pin should be cen-tered laterally. The condylar guidance in-clination should be very similar.

4. If a large difference is recorded (more than 6° to 7°), another bite should be taken and the recordings verified.

5. Set the lateral condylar inclination (see *Setting of the Lateral Condylar In-clination*, p. 118).

Setting of Horizontal Condylar Inclination Without Protrusive Check Bite

In some instances a protrusive registra-tion may not be available, but a method can be used to set the condylar inclination in most instances. Also, the method can be used to cross check the accuracy of the protrusive registration. A knowledge of some aspects of the contact relations in the mouth is necessary.

1. Loosen the condylar inclination thumbnuts and make certain the condylar elements move freely in the slot. Set the condylar inclination to 20° to 25°.

2. Raise the incisal pin out of contact with the table.

3. Place the casts together so that cus-pids in *right* lateral protrusive have con-tact (Fig. 7–32A,B,C). Adjust the left con-dylar inclination if necessary to obtain contact of cuspids. Move the *left* condylar inclination backward and forward until the

position is found in which the cuspids on the *right* are just out of contact (Fig. 7–33A,B,C).

4. The left condylar inclination may be close to zero (Fig. 7–33C) or have a nega-tive value. Then bring the right cuspids *just* back together by changing the *left* condylar inclination. Increase the horizon-tal condylar inclination until light contact is made on the balancing side.

5. At this point minimum condylar in-clination has been reached.* This proce-dure can be used only when posterior teeth are present. It can be used also as a check upon the correctness of a protrusive check bite (see Unit 8). Use lateral incisors or bicuspids if necessary if cuspid contacts are inadequate.

6. Repeat procedure 3 using a left later-al protrusive position and adjust the right condylar inclination.

7. Repeat procedure 3 with the casts in the straight protrusive, incisal edge-to-edge position. Relate to posterior protru-sive contacts or protrusive interferences or both, involving posterior teeth that pre-vent occlusion of anterior teeth.

Setting of the Lateral Condylar Inclination

1. Utilizing the formula (Fig. 2–4) on the bottom of the articulator, calculate the lat-eral condylar guide setting bilaterally (H = horizontal condylar guide setting, L = lateral).

2. Release the set screw on the posterior of each vertical axis and rotate until the calculated setting is reached, then secure the set screw.

---

*Note: At this time ask the question: Does the patient have left balancing side contact? This infor-mation should have been obtained during the clinical examination. If the answer is yes, there is balancing contact, the condylar inclination need only be adjust-ed slightly to ensure contact of facets of wear on the left side. If in making balancing contact there is right working side disclusion of the cuspids, the change is too much or a left balancing side interference is present in the mouth. This information also should have been obtained at the time of the examination. If the answer is that there is no contact on the balancing side in the mouth, then the clinician must decide on one of two approaches: have the patient return for a protrusive check bite, or utilize the balancing side contact as a "fudge factor" to ensure that no balancing interference will be formed during waxing of a res-toration.

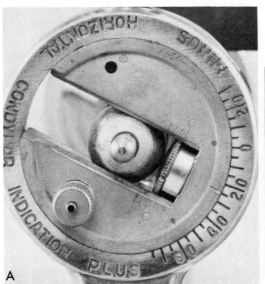

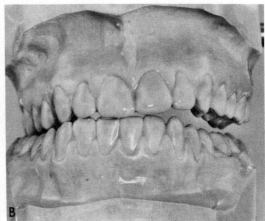

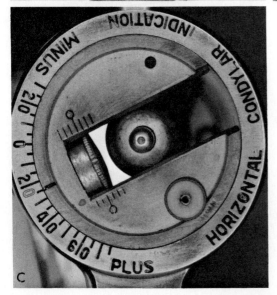

Figure 7–32. Setting horizontal condylar inclination without protrusive check bite (see text).

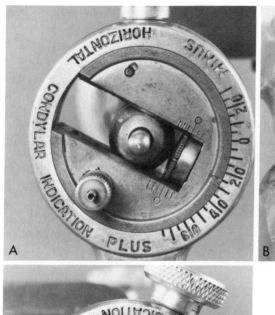

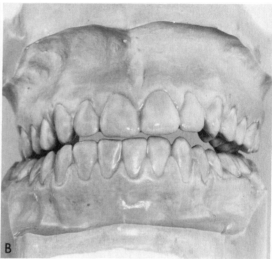

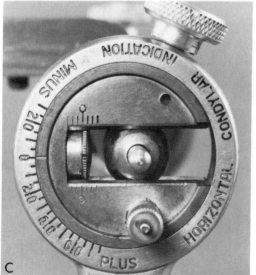

Figure 7–33. Setting horizontal condylar inclination without protrusive check bite (see text).

Unit 7 Exercises

1. Why is it necessary to analyze articulated casts?

   a. _____

   b. _____

2. Holding the casts statically in the straight protrusive excursion, change the horizontal condylar guidance from 50° to 0°, observing the changing relationship of the molar teeth.
   a. Briefly describe this change.

   _____

   _____

   b. What effect could be seen if restorations were fabricated with the condylar inclinations arbitrarily set steeper than that given by a protrusive wax record?

   _____

   _____

3. Holding the casts statically in a straight left lateral excursion (mandibular and maxillary cusp tips on the left working side in end-to-end contact), change the right side balancing condylar inclination *from 50° to 0°*.
   a. Briefly describe the changing relationship of the molar teeth on the balancing side.

   _____

   _____

   b. On the working side (condylar elements against centric stops).

   _____

   _____

   c. If the horizontal condylar inclination on the balancing side is arbitrarily set more shallow than that of the patient, does this ensure more clearance or less clearance between cusps on the balancing side of the patient?

   _____

   _____

4. Holding the casts statically in a lateral protrusive excursion (between straight protrusive and straight lateral), describe for the working and balancing sides: (1) the result of changing the condylar inclination on the working side from 50° to 0°, and (2) the result of changing the condylar inclination on the balancing side from 50° to 0°.

   a. Describe the change on the working side for (1) and (2):

_____

_____

_____

_____

   b. Describe the change on the balancing side for (1) and (2):

_____

_____

_____

_____

5. With the horizontal condylar inclination set at 64° and the lateral condylar inclination set at 20°, simulate a right lateral excursion. With the articulator in this position, change the lateral condylar inclination from 20° and 0° on the balancing side.

   a. What happens to the space between the condylar ball and the shaft housing on the working side?

_____

_____

Duplicate the situation while holding the upper member of the articulator toward the working side.

   b. Describe the relationship of the condylar element to the shaft housing.

_____

_____

   c. What effect might be expected on the occlusion if the articulator is not manipulated properly? (Pushing the upper member toward the balancing side is considered correct.)

_____

_____

   d. What effect might be seen on a full crown restoration by not recording a lateral condylar inclination similar to the Bennett angle of the patient?

_____

_____

6. If the incisal guidance of the articulator does not duplicate the guidance provided by the patient, it becomes an end controlling factor of the occlusion. What would the consequence be of fabricating posterior restorations with too deep an incisal guidance?

_____

_____

7. What errors are visible in Figure 7–34?

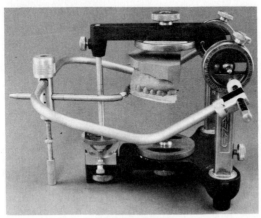

Figure 7–34.

_____

_____

8. Of what value is the mounting of casts by simulation methods?

_____

9. The more anterior the position of the mandible is for a protrusive check bite registration, the greater the possibility for error in the condylar inclination

due to _____ ; the less anterior the position, the greater the

possibility of not having a distinct difference between _____

_____

10. Relative to the setting of the condylar inclination, what do the facets of wear suggest in Figure 7–35?

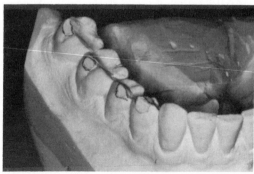

Figure 7–35.

_____

_____

11. At what value is the condylar inclination set for in mounting the mandibular cast in simulated centric relation and with a check bite?

_____

12. The greater the discrepancy between centric occlusion and centric relation, the greater the influence by the condylar inclination. How does this influence the use of the articulator during waxing restorations?

_____

Unit 7 Test

1. The most accurate method of locating the true hinge axis is:

   a. hinge axis locator
   b. simple face bow
   c. ear piece face bow
   d. centric relation check bite
   e. none of the above

2. An arbitrary hinge axis is located on the patient by measurement:

   a. using a kinematic face bow
   b. ~13 mm anterior to tragus
   c. a and b
   d. by an ear piece face bow (Hanau)
   e. a, b, and d

3. An ear piece face bow (Hanau) locates the arbitrary hinge axis:

    a. "automatically"
    b. by measurement
    c. 13 mm anterior to the tragus
    d. with an error of ± .5 mm
    e. none of the above

4. The condylar inclination setting to use the simple face bow must be:

    a. 0
    b. 20
    c. 50
    d. 70
    e. none of the above

5. When the condylar inclination is in the right position for use with the ear piece face bow, the distance from the articulator axle and the ear piece pin is:

    a. 10 mm
    b. 11 mm
    c. 12 mm
    d. 13 mm
    e. none of the above

6. In using the ear piece face bow, the incisal edges of the maxillary anterior teeth should be what distance above the surface of the lower member of the articulator?

    a. 50 mm
    b. 54 mm
    c. 58 mm
    d. 62 mm
    e. none of the above

7. If no face bow is used to mount the maxillary cast on the articulator, what is the most important principle to follow in arbitrarily mounting the maxillary cast?

    a. maximize tooth guidance
    b. maximize incisal guidance
    c. maximize horizontal condylar guidance
    d. maximize lateral condylar guidance
    e. none of the above

8. If no centric relation check bite is used to mount the mandibular cast, how may a simulated centric relation mounting be obtained?

    a. mount the mandibular cast in centric occlusion with PR adjustment moved clockwise
    b. mount the mandibular cast in centric occlusion with a shim inserted between condylar elements and condylar stops
    c. a and b
    d. mount the mandibular cast in centric occlusion with PR adjusted to minus zero
    e. a, b, and d

9. If no protrusive check bite is available, what clinical information is necessary to set the condylar inclination?

   a. balancing contact
   b. balancing interferences
   c. a and b
   d. angle of eminentia
   e. a, b, and d

10. In setting the horizontal condylar inclination without a protrusive check bite as well as checking the accuracy of the inclination set with a protrusive check bite, the smallest condylar inclination is set by:

   a. balancing contacts
   b. lateral protrusive contacts
   c. a and b
   d. incisal edge contacts
   e. a, b, and d

11. In Figure 7–36 the upper cast will (move upward, move downward, not move) when the condylar inclination is moved as in (1) or in (2):

   a. move downward, (1)
   b. move upward, (2)
   c. move upward, (1)
   d. move downward, (2)
   e. not move, (1) or (2)

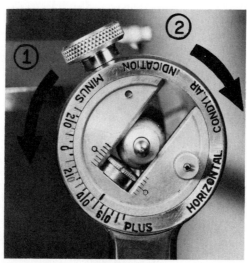

Figure 7–36.

12. In a simulated centric relation mounting of the mandibular cast, which of the following is (are) true:

   a. cast positioned in centric occlusion
   b. condylar stop set counterclockwise
   c. a and b
   d. condylar inclination set at zero
   e. a, b, and d

Unit 8

Evaluation of Mounted Casts and Potential Errors in Mounting Procedures

After the casts have been mounted and functional records secured, the articulation must be evaluated. Because of common errors in mounting the mandibular cast, this step should be checked immediately before proceeding to a complete evaluation of the mounted casts.

A number of potential errors in the mounting of casts may prevent proper articulation of the casts; some are inherent in the instruments, others are due to human error. Both may be minimized by an understanding of the source of errors.

INTRODUCTION: UNIT OBJECTIVES AND READING

The objective of this unit is to present methods for evaluating the adequacy of the mounting of casts on the articulator, and to describe some of the sources of potential error in the instruments and procedures.

A. Objectives
1. Be able to identify steps in evaluating the correctness of mounted casts.
2. Be able to discuss the nature of the problem in incorrectly mounted casts.
3. Be able to identify the potential

errors in instruments used: articulator and face bow.
4. Discuss the potential errors in the centric relation check bite.

B. Reading (optional)
Schuyler, C. H.: Occlusion in restorative dentistry. Ohio Dent. J. March 1963.

EVALUATION OF MOUNTING

A quick evaluation of the adequacy of a centric relation mounting of the mandibular cast involves first the determination of whether or not the casts can be articulated in centric occlusion. This can be done without resorting to a split cast technique of mounting the maxillary cast. Thus the first step in the mounting evaluation is to determine the adequacy of centric occlusion stops: visually at first and then with shim stock. Except for potential errors discussed previously, the centric stops present in the mouth at the examination should be present on the articulated casts.

Centric Stops

The location of stops and their presence may be determined with 28 gauge green

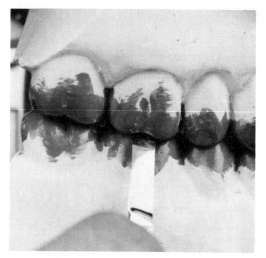

Figure 8–1. Centric stops. Very thin shim stock (0.0005 in) is used to determine the presence or absence of centric stops.

sheet inlay wax and 5 ten thousand shim stock* (Fig. 8–1); however, a visual test should be carried out first. This is done by loosening the thumbnut holding the maxillary cast while keeping the maxillary cast seated firmly in maximum intercuspation. With the two casts held firmly together, the thumbnut is tightened. As the thumbnut is tightened fully, the maxillary cast should not come out of maximum contact with the mandibular cast. If there is separation or a lateral shift, the mounting of the mandibular cast may be incorrect due to (1) incorrect CR checkbite, (2) failure to seat casts correctly in CR checkbite, (3) both 1 and 2, (4) the condylar setting is

---

*Artus Corp., Englewood, NJ 07631

incorrect due to a faulty protrusive bite record, (5) the condylar path is curved, or (6) the face bow transfer may be incorrect, especially the angulation of the plane of occlusion. If the casts are placed securely into the centric relation check bite and the thumbnut is loosened, the maxillary cast should not come out of the check bite when the thumbnut is tightened. If so, the mandibular cast should be remounted accurately in the check bite. The most probable cause of a shift in the cast out of centric occlusion is incorrect CR check bite.

Working, Balancing, and Protrusive Relations

If facets of wear are present on the casts, contacts involving these facets should be possible if such contact relations are present in the mouth (Fig. 8–2). All such contact relations should be evaluated, especially lateral protrusive. If in lateral protrusive contact positions there is a lack of contacts involving facets of wear, the condylar guidance inclination should be adjusted in order to obtain the contacts of facets of wear. Correlate occlusal examination with the presence of balancing, working, and protrusive interferences.

Straight Working. There should be no effect on contact relations on the working side with changes of condylar inclination. Working contacts involving facets of wear should be present if present in the mouth and if balancing interferences are not present. If there is a significant discrepancy between centric occlusion and centric relation, there will be a change in working side contacts if the condylar inclination is

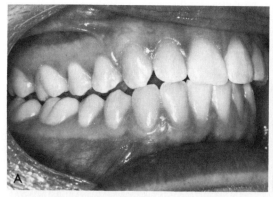
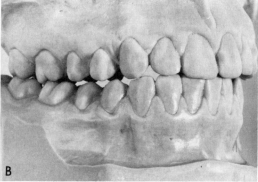

Figure 8–2. Occlusal contacts. *A,* cuspid and molar contact relations in patient should be duplicated on mounted casts as shown in *B.* All other contacts should be tested in balancing and protrusive.

changed with the condylar element in centric occlusion on the working side.

Lateral Protrusive. Place the casts in lateral protrusive so that the cuspids are in end-to-end contact on the working side. Then change the condylar guidance from 0° to 50° to 0°, observing the relationship of cuspids and balancing side relations. With the cuspids just in end-to-end contact because of the balancing side condylar guidance setting, the balancing side relations should be the same as in the mouth. Balancing side contacts involving facets of wear should match.

Protrusive Contact Relations. With the casts in protrusive relations, the movement patterns involving incisal and cuspid wear should be capable of being duplicated on the articulated casts.

Slide in Centric

The magnitude and direction of the slide in centric should correspond with that in the mouth.

Premature Contacts

The location of premature contacts in centric relation should be marked in the mouth with articulating paper and checked with 28 gauge green sheet inlay wax. 28 gauge wax should also be used to check the location of premature contacts on the articulated casts. The location in the mouth and on the casts should be the same. Thus when the wax is placed in the mouth and the patient is guided into centric relation closure to contact, the perforation caused by the initial contact should be the same as when the procedure is repeated with the articulated casts.

POTENTIAL ERRORS IN MOUNTING CASTS IN AN ARTICULATOR

The potential errors to be discussed here are related to a semi-adjustable articulator and more specifically to the Hanau H2 and H2–PR. However, many of these errors are common to many other articulators and to the procedures involved.

The possibility of making errors in the mounting of casts may be: (1) inherent in *method* (true hinge versus arbitrary hinge axis) and in devices (articulators and face bows); (2) caused by improper manipulation of material (wax, plaster) used to register the mandibular position in centric relation; and (3) caused by the difficulty involved in the manipulation of the mandible into centric relation (operator inexperience, the presence of temporomandibular joint and/or muscle dysfunction or a combination of these).

Inherent Errors

Hinge Axis. A simple face bow utilizes the arbitrary hinge axis, not the "true" hinge axis obtained by a kinematic face bow. The error involved is minimized by having the interocclusal record of wax in centric relation very thin — less than 3 mm.

Figure 8–3 simulates the anteroposterior error (about 0.2 mm) at the second molar that occurs with an interocclusal centric relation record of a thickness of about 3 mm taken when there is a 5-mm discrepancy between the true hinge axis and the arbitrary hinge axis. R_1 is the radius for the true hinge axis and R_2 the radius for the arbitrary hinge axis. The error would be hypothetically zero if the thickness of the CR check bite were zero.

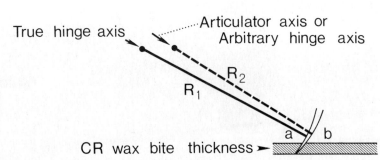

Figure 8–3. Hinge axis error. Potential error of using arbitrary versus true hinge axis (see text).

Third Point of Reference. With the ear piece face bow, the third point of the reference should be at the lower notch on the incisal pin (~58 mm from the top surface of the articulator's base). At that point the A/B difference will be essentially zero. A, the support pin for the ear face bow, is ~0.046 mm below and ~12 mm posterior to the articulator axis, B. Raising or lowering the third point of reference with the ear rod face bow results in error (Fig. 8–4), both anteroposterior and vertical.

Condylar Path. There are two basic problems commonly discussed in connection with potential errors involving the use of a semi-adjustable articulator such as the Hanau H2 or H2–PR: condylar guidance and Bennett shift.

Condylar Guidance. The condylar guidance (slot) is straight while the actual path of the condyle may be curved or zigzag. This may produce an error of practical clinical significance. In determining the effect of a straight slot on the mounting of casts, it is necessary to consider (1) the position of the condyle in centric relation and centric occlusion, (2) the position dictated by the straight slot and condylar guidance inclination on the articulator, and (3) the position of the condylar element dictated by the casts in centric occlusion. The error from a curved condylar path is usually small compared to the magnitude of the error that is possible and often occurs to some degree in obtaining the CR wax bite, i.e., the interocclusal record of centric relation.

If casts are mounted on an articulator (H2–PR) using a centric relation check bite, the condylar elements of the articulator should rest against the centric stops when the casts are in centric relation. With the centric stop unlocked and the maxillary cast moved into centric occlusion, any change in the condylar guidance setting will raise or lower the maxillary cast. Any movement from centric relation to centric

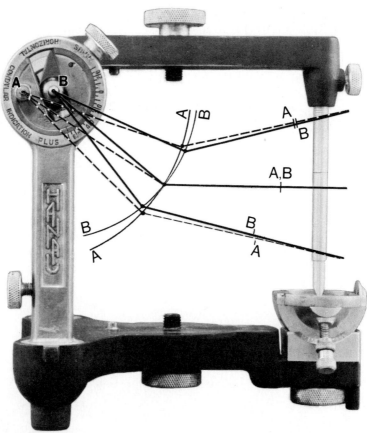

Figure 8–4. Ear piece face bow error. Potential error of Hanau ear piece face bow related to third point of reference. (See text.)

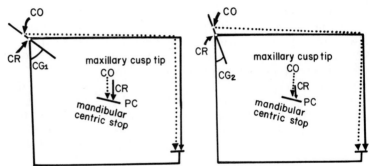

Figure 8–5. Condylar guide error. Potential error involving discrepancy between path of condyle and condylar guide of articulator (see text). $\leftarrow\cdots$ indicates maxillary cusp tip contact. CG is condylar guidance inclination of articulator. PC is the plane of the centric stop.

occlusion will result in an elevation of the maxillary cast for any positive angulation of the condylar guidance.

For a condylar inclination of 30°, a movement of the condylar element of 1 mm from centric relation to centric occlusion will cause the maxillary cast to be elevated about one ten-thousandth of an inch at the second molar. For a condylar inclination of 60°, the elevation will be about 2 ten-thousandths of an inch. Our shim stock for testing centric stops is 5 ten-thousandths of an inch in thickness.

There should be no loss of centric stops between centric relation and centric occlusion, but any movement beyond centric occlusion will lead to *disclusion* (loss of contact) of centric stops of posterior teeth. Maintenance of centric stops is an important reason for obtaining the proper centric relation position, including the proper distance from centric occlusion to centric relation.

Figure 8–5 is a schematic representation of an articulator set at two different condylar guidance inclinations (CG_1 and CG_2) for the same set of mounted casts. With the correct condylar inclination (CG_1), there will be contact of the supporting cusp tips (only one maxillary cusp tip shown at arrow is used here) in centric relation and centric occlusion, and between centric relation and centric occlusion. However, if the condylar guidance inclination is incorrectly set (CG_2*), there will be no contact of the supporting cusp with the centric stop in centric occlusion; only in centric relation will there be contact. A curved condylar path could produce the same error, but because of the common and

more gross error to be discussed relative to the CR check bite and the cushioning effect of the temporomandibular joint disc, the curved condylar path error is not a common problem. There is also a correlation between the inclination of the plane of occlusion, the radius of the curve of Spee, and the magnitude of the error produced by an incorrect condylar inclination setting. The more divergent the plane of occlusion and the condylar inclination, the greater the magnitude of error if centric relation to centric occlusion is large (> than 1 mm). The shorter the radius of the curve of Spee, the less the magnitude of the error is likely to be.

In Figure 8–6, CP shows a theoretical curved condylar path and the condylar guidance CG1 set from a protrusive (PI) check bite with the mandible too far forward. CG2 is the condylar guidance set

---

*CG_2 is assumed to be incorrectly set for demonstration purposes — proof is the absence of contact at centric occlusion.

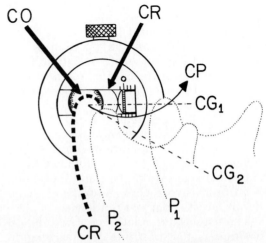

Figure 8–6. Condylar guide error. Potential error due to curved path of condyle and straight slot of articulator condylar guide. (See text.)

with a much shorter protrusive (P2) check bite, but incorporating the path from centric relation to centric occlusion. The Hanau H2–PR as well as other similar articulators does not have provisions for curved condylar paths.

Inasmuch as the horizontal condylar guidance is set by two points (protrusive and centric relation/centric occlusion) the position of the condylar element at centric occlusion is important since the casts may not occlude (make contact) in the molar region if the condylar guidance is incorrect, especially with a curved condylar path. However, from a practical standpoint the presence or absence of posterior contacts can be checked on the articulator. Those centric stops present in the patient should be present on the articulator. If they are absent on the articulator, the most likely error is in the centric relation check bite.

There is less possibility of error from a curved path with a good protrusive record and when attention is paid to the presence or absence of centric stops in centric occlusion. When an experienced operator takes a centric relation record and has an optimal condylar guidance but cannot get the casts together in centric occlusion, there is the possibility that the condylar path is curved and the condylar guidance cannot be set properly. This problem is most likely to occur when there is an extensive slide in centric and a curved condylar path is present.

For the inexperienced operator it is sometimes advocated that the mandibular cast be mounted in centric occlusion directly (without a centric occlusion wax check bite) and the PR adjustment be set back to zero. (It must be recognized that the true centric relation position is not known, and adjustment of restorations from centric occlusion to centric relation may be necessary or contact may not exist from centric occlusion to centric relation position.) The primary reason for this procedure is the inability of the inexperienced operator to (1) take an interocclusal centric relation record, (2) evaluate for centric occlusion contacts properly, and (3) obtain a good protrusive record. Another explanation is curved condylar guidance.

The use of a simulated centric relation position is no substitute for learning to obtain an optimal protrusive check bite

and a precise centric relation wax record, and to evaluate for the adequacy of centric stops. If an adequate mounting can be obtained for diagnostic purposes, one can be obtained for restorative procedures insofar as centric occlusion centric stops are concerned. When it appears that a centric relation check bite cannot be obtained because of operator inexperience or muscle hypertonicity, the casts can be mounted in centric occlusion with the PR adjustment set for a simulated centric relation, provided the limitations of the simulated centric relation position are understood.

Bennett Movement and Side Shift. Medial and anterior movement of the balancing side condyle (Bennett movement) is simulated as an angle on the articulator. All of the movement is a progressive side shift on the Hanau H2–PR; there is no significant component of immediate side shift. The theoretical potential for error from failure to measure an immediate side shift has been discussed in relation to so-called condylar determinants of occlusion.

The movement of the working side condyle in both the vertical and horizontal planes is demonstrated elsewhere. The Hanau H2–PR simulates only one type of movement, which can be seen by visual inspection of the condylar shaft on the working side. Potential errors are also discussed in relation to condylar determinants of occlusion.

Interocclusal Records

Centric Relation. As indicated in Figure 8–7A, CB_1 is an accurate centric relation check bite. With the mandibular cast mounted using CB_1 there would be simultaneous contact of all centric stops (arrows with c in Figure 8–7B) because of the hinge axis closure (HAC). However, if there is an error as in CB_2 (Fig. 8–7C), caused by either a check bite not being taken on the patient's hinge axis (HA) or the patient's hinge axis not being the same as the articulator axis (AA), the occlusal surfaces (OS_1 and OS_2) will not contact simultaneously but will often contact only in the anterior (Fig. 8–7D). This error often occurs because of insufficiently softened wax or improper manipulation of the man-

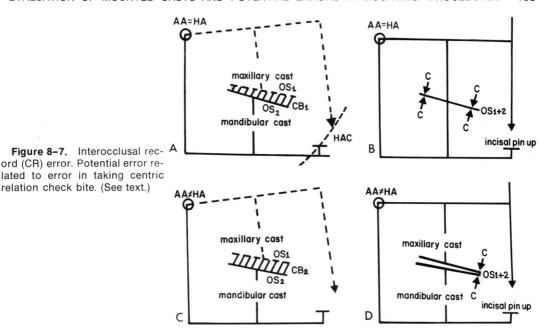

Figure 8–7. Interocclusal record (CR) error. Potential error related to error in taking centric relation check bite. (See text.)

dible in centric relation, or because face bow transfer is not representative of patient's hinge axis (AA ≠ HA), or a combination of these factors.

Protrusive. The protrusive check bite used to set the condylar guidance on the Hanau H2–PR articulator requires that the protrusive movement be straight forward for a limited distance and that both condylar guidances will be the same. The error associated with a curved path and the protrusive movement exceeding 4 to 5 mm has already been discussed. Also, if the movement is not straight forward, the condylar guidance settings may differ easily more than 10 degrees. If the protrusive record is not correctly taken, the errors that can occur when restorations are placed in the mouth include (1) premature contacts in centric relation and centric occlusion, (2) open contacts in centric relation and between centric occlusion and centric relation, and (3) faulty contact relations in lateral protrusive, viz., balancing side interferences.

A good check on the adequacy of the setting of the condylar guidance inclination can be done without the patient being present. However, a comparison of the occlusal relation in the patient and on the

articulator is the only satisfactory method if the occlusal examination is adequate, as indicated in Unit 6.

The use of an interocclusal record on the balancing side as well as on the working side will provide a check on the protrusive record and condylar inclination. Keep in mind that the Hanau H2–PR does not accept lateral check bites. However, the 15° setting of the lateral condylar guidance will approximate the average lateral guidance and the wax record can be used with some degree of accuracy.

In summary, limitations of such devices as semi-adjustable articulators and face bows are counteracted or minimized to one extent or another by use of various procedures or more complex instruments or both, viz., functionally generated path procedures or "fully" adjustable articulators or both. In any case the accurate recording of centric relation is a procedure that must be mastered at some point. (The use of pantographics or stereographics to obtain border movements and to program fully adjustable articulators, as well as the use of nonarticulator instruments such as the Gnathic Relator, are not necessary for the vast majority of cases. Their use will not be described here.)

Unit 8 Exercises

1. What is the first indication that the mounting of a mandibular cast in centric relation is incorrect?

   _____

   _____

2. What may be the cause of disclusion of cuspids in a lateral protrusive position?

   _____

   _____

3. Why is the third point of reference more important with use of the ear piece face bow than with the use of the simple face bow?

   _____

   _____

4. What would the potential error be from using a simple face bow if the thickness of the centric relation check bite was hypothetically zero?

   _____

   _____

5. What establishes the optimal amount of protrusion for a protrusive check bite?

   _____

   _____

6. Assume that your mounting is such that all centric stops are correct, premature contacts are in the right place, and all contacts made in mandibular excursions in the mouth can be made on the mounted casts. What clinical problems may be present?

   _____

   _____

7. If casts are mounted incorrectly in centric relation so that posterior centric stops are missing on some teeth, how may the error be corrected?

   _____

   _____

8. What are the potential errors associated with using a simulated centric relation mounting for waxing restorations to be used on patients?

   _____

   _____

9. On an arcon articulator such as the Denar or Whip-Mix, the upper member rests on the condylar elements but can be removed. If the upper member guidance are not maintained in contact with the condylar elements during waxing posterior restorations, which error may occur?

_____

_____

10. What is the significance of absent lateral contacts on the casts in waxing a restoration? Contacts in working when there are no contacts in the mouth?

_____

_____

Unit 8 Test

1. The most common error in mounting casts in centric relation in a semi-adjustable articulator results from:

   a. incorrect centric relation check bite
   b. curved articulator condylar guide
   c. use of arbitrary hinge axis
   d. incorrect setting of third point of reference for face bow
   e. none of the above

2. A common cause of an incorrect centric relation check bite is:

   a. failure to use thoroughly softened wax for the check bite
   b. muscle hypertonicity
   c. a and b
   d. patient not trained in procedure
   e. a, b, and d

3. If facets of wear do not occlude in a working relation but do in the mouth, the problem may be:

   a. incorrect condylar setting
   b. articulator design may be inadequate
   c. discrepancy between proper plane of occlusion setting and condylar inclination
   d. incorrect centric relation check bite
   e. all of the above

4. If it is found that there is an absence of centric stops on the molars just after mounting the mandibular cast in centric relation on an articulator, the first step should be:

   a. retake the CR check bite
   b. loosen the maxillary cast, occlude in CR bite, and tighten the thumbnut of the maxillary cast to check if the cast maintains contacts in check bite
   c. decrease condylar inclination to minus zero
   d. increase condylar inclination to 50°
   e. remove maxillary cast and remount

5. The third reference point is more important for the Hanau ear piece face bow than for the non ear piece face bow because:

   a. the ear piece does not rest on the transverse axis of the articulator
   b. the third point of reference for the non ear piece face bow reference can be set at any point without error
   c. the non ear rod face bow is not related to the hinge axis
   d. the ear piece face bow is inherently more accurate
   e. none of the above

6. If a molar full crown is waxed to contact in centric occlusion when centric occlusion stops are absent due to an incorrect centric relation mounting:

   a. the crown will be "high" in the mouth in centric occlusion
   b. "high" in working
   c. "high" in balancing
   d. "high" in protrusive
   e. all of the above

7. Which of the following is most accurate for obtaining a centric relation mounting of the mandibular cast?

   a. use of PR adjustment
   b. use of shim between condylar element and condylar stop
   c. use of CR check bite
   d. use of hinge axis locator
   e. none of the above

8. If the condylar inclination is different by more than about 7° between sides, the most common cause is:

   a. face bow positioned incorrectly
   b. protrusive check bite taken too far forward
   c. not enough protrusion in taking check bite
   d. protrusion not straight in taking check bite
   e. none of the above

9. In order to properly check the condylar setting from a protrusive check bite it is necessary to have information from the oral examination. What should be known?

   a. balancing side contacts or not
   b. edge-to-edge incisor contacts or not
   c. balancing and working interferences or not
   d. protrusive interferences or not
   e. none of the above

10. If casts are mounted in centric occlusion rather than centric relation and the condylar elements of the Hanau H2 articulator are against the condylar stops, the element:

    a. will rest on the hinge axis of the articulator
    b. will change in position with changing condylar inclinations
    c. a and b
    d. will move into a retrusive position
    e. a, b, and d

Unit 9

Occlusal Adjustment

An occlusal adjustment is indicated for the treatment of functional disturbances and is done before comprehensive restorative procedures. The method of adjustment has been described in detail elsewhere. A brief review of the procedure will be done as it relates to an occlusal adjustment of the casts that were mounted in a simulated centric relation in Units 6 and 7. The adjusted casts can be used for waxing of a splint in Unit 11. Unadjusted casts will be used in Unit 10, *Waxing Functional Occlusion–1*. The objective of this unit is to describe some of the general principles for an occlusal adjustment.

Only a sharp knife, shim stock, and articulating paper are needed for the occlusal adjustment of the casts.

INTRODUCTION: UNIT OBJECTIVES AND READINGS

During an occlusal adjustment decisions on where and how much to grind (adjust) must be made constantly. Without a knowledge of the goals of, the sequence of steps in, and rules for the adjustment, it would become a hopeless procedure. Several behavioral objectives are suggested.
A. Objectives
  1. Be able to name the steps in occlusal adjustment on casts.
  2. Be able to give the criteria for completion of an occlusal adjustment.
  3. Be able to list the principles and rules for an occlusal adjustment.
B. Readings (optional)
  Ramfjord, S. R. and Ash, M. M., Jr.: Occlusion. Philadelphia, W. B. Saunders Co., 1971 (Chapter 13).

Schuyler, C. H.: Fundamental principles in the correction of occlusal disharmony, natural and artificial. J.A.D.A. pp. 1193–1202, July, 1935.

STEPS IN THE OCCLUSAL ADJUSTMENT ON CASTS

Step 1. Paint the occlusal surfaces of the casts with Die-Spacer.* Determine and record the centric stops (Fig. 9–1). The incisal pin should be in contact with the incisal table in centric occlusion.
Step 2. Do the occlusal adjustment in centric relation (Fig. 9–2). With the upper member locked in centric relation, the pin will not be in contact with the incisal table until the occlusal interference in centric relation is removed.
Step 3. Continue the occlusal adjustment for working and balancing (Fig. 9–3).
Step 4. Complete the occlusal adjustment for protrusive and lateral protrusive.
Step 5. Complete the occlusal adjustment by smoothing the adjusted areas. The incisal pin should be in contact with the incisal table in centric occlusion and centric relation.

OCCLUSAL ADJUSTMENT: THEORETICAL CONSIDERATIONS

A tendency is often present when doing an occlusal adjustment on casts to grind

---

*Die-Spacer, Protex-M, 735 Ocean Ave., Brooklyn, NY, 11226.

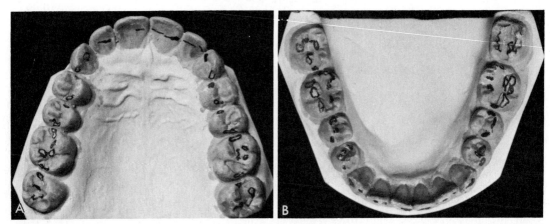

Figure 9–1. Centric stops. Centric stops are seldom single contacts in the natural dentition. *A* and *B*, primary and secondary contacts on maxillary and mandibular teeth.

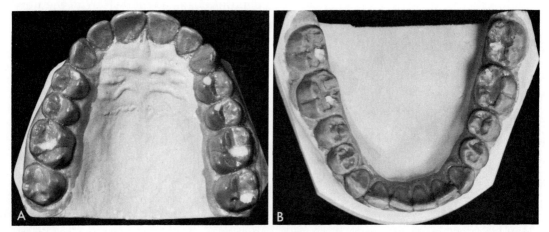

Figure 9–2. Occlusal adjustment in centric relation. *A, B*, completion of occlusal adjustment on maxillary and mandibular casts. Adjustment of buccal inclines of lingual cusps of the mandibular molars was done for premature contacts involving the axial surfaces and cusp ridges of the maxillary molars.

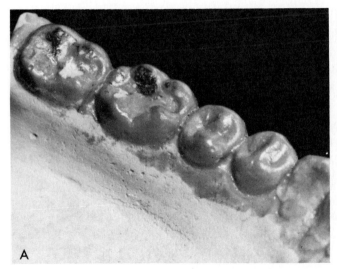
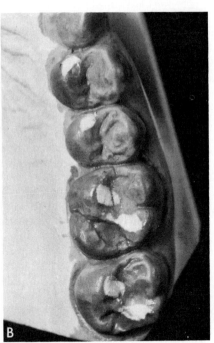

Figure 9–3. Occlusal adjustment for working, balancing, and protrusive interferences. Occlusal interferences were present only on balancing side in right working movement. *A,* balancing interferences before occlusal adjustment; *B,* after removal of interferences. No adjustment of the mandibular molars was necessary to eliminate the balancing interferences.

excessively, almost as if "balanced occlusion" were the goal of an occlusal adjustment. However, the adjustment should not be directed toward a balanced occlusion, group function, a "cuspid protected occlusion," "point centric," or toward any restriction on mandibular position or movement — it should be directed toward eliminating interferences to mandibular closure and smooth gliding contact movements.

Adjustment on Casts

There are some obvious visual advantages to doing an occlusal adjustment on casts, but the adjustment in the mouth cannot be based on what is accomplished on the casts without reservation because of the limitations on the articular simulation of mandibular movements. The detection of occlusal balancing and working side interferences in the mouth is often difficult because it is necessary to depend on digital palpation to determine heavy contact or tooth movement or both. When a balancing interference causes disclusion on the working side, this may be seen easily on mounted casts. However, in the mouth, under heavy function, a tooth having the balancing interference may move and disclusion on the working side may

not occur. This does not occur with casts. Thus the detection of balancing (or working) side interferences in the mouth requires tactile as well as visual sense.

On the working side the contact of one or two teeth is sometimes considered to be an interference, and interference to multiple contacts in working. However, contacts on individual teeth are not considered to be interferences unless the involved teeth have increased mobility or loss of support or both and it is desired to distribute occlusal forces over more teeth. Gross removal of tooth structure to obtain multiple contacts is contraindicated.

As balancing side interferences are reduced, increased contact may occur on the working side (bicuspid, cuspid, lateral incisors and/or central incisors). A reduction of the cuspid to increase posterior contacts can result in excessive contacts on the bicuspid to central incisor teeth. A reduction of the maxillary cuspid and incisors to increase posterior contacts or promote group function is contraindicated.

Value of Adjusting Study Casts

Beyond its function in teaching, the value of doing an occlusal adjustment on study casts in the clinical situation depends upon several factors: (1) the need for doing the adjustment on stone casts prior to treatment of the patient, (2) the extent to which the articulator can duplicate jaw movements, and (3) how well the occlusal relations of the patient have been "captured" and transferred to the articulator.

After the principles of the occlusal adjustment are learned, it is seldom necessary to do an occlusal adjustment on study casts. However, it is sometimes impossible to predict accurately how much tooth structure may be safely removed in the adjustment and how the adjustment should relate to a restorative problem, or both these factors, without doing the adjustment on stone casts. Furthermore, not all occlusal problems can be solved by an occlusal adjustment, viz., food impaction caused by "opening up" of contact may be due to a new restoration with inadequate occlusal relations. After a tooth has drifted distally and interproximal contact has been lost, a new restoration and adequate occlusal relations may be the only solution for food impaction. Certainly, the use of dental tape or floss is only symptomatic treatment for most cases of food impaction. Permanent treatment involves occlusal therapy. Often the exact nature of the occlusal problem can be determined only by study casts and an occlusal adjustment. The need for doing an occlusal adjustment on casts must be determined for each patient.

The Hanau H2–PR articulator is adequate for an occlusal adjustment of study casts. Its limitations on duplication of mandibular movements can best be appreciated by observing contact relations in the patient and on the study casts. All articulators have limitations, some more than others. To use a fully adjustment articulator for study casts would be an unwarranted expenditure of time and effort. In most instances a semi-adjustable articulator is very adequate.

Adjustment Decisions

Decisions must be made constantly during the occlusal adjustment: whether to grind on maxillary or mandibular teeth, to grind away a centric stop, or to grind to obtain more working contacts. A general rule is to grind away from function — that is, away from cusp ridges that function in

working or away from centric stops and buccal axial surfaces that function in working. For example, where does one grind when there is an extensive balancing interference involving the lingual cusp of No. 3 (maxillary right first molar) and the distal cusp of No. 30 (mandibular right first molar) if a supporting cusp has to be eliminated? In this case the grinding involves the maxillary lingual cusp. Because of the number of centric stops on the molars, the loss of the stop on the right maxillary first molar (No. 3) is more desirable for stability and function than the loss of the supporting cusp stop on the right first mandibular molar (No. 30). In some instances it may be possible to adjust the occlusion on both No. 3 and No. 30 without losing the centric stop of the mesial lingual cusp of No. 3.

An occlusal interference on the bicuspids often involves the mesial lingual cusp ridge of the maxillary first premolar and the distal cusp ridge of the mandibular premolar. The grinding should be done on the mesial cusp ridge until the centric stop on the maxillary premolar is in jeopardy, then the distal cusp ridge of the mandibular premolar should be ground. If the premature contact in centric relation involves the distal slope of the triangular ridge or transverse ridge, grinding may be done here in addition to the lingual cusp ridge of the maxillary premolar if it does not undermine the cusp ridge or result in a step between centric relation and centric occlusion. The decision on where to grind must be tempered by the need for occlusal stability and function.

Teeth to be Restored

When an occlusal adjustment is being done in the immediate preparatory phase of restorative dental treatment, it is sometimes thought that the normal rules for adjustment dealing with occlusal stability and conservation of tooth structure need not be followed. This approach should not be used on the patient and not on study casts until the best course of action has been determined. From the standpoint of the adjustment of the patient, the teeth may shift and extrude before the actual restorative phase is undertaken. From the standpoint of the study casts, the opposing occlusion must be compatible with the predicted restored occlusion.

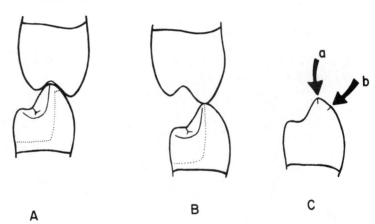

Figure 9–4. Occlusal adjustment and margins of restorations (see text).

A   B   C

In the event that the continued adjustment of a tooth could result in excessive loss of its structure, the adjustment should be completed on its antagonist. However, in some instances the occlusion of both teeth may be so dysfunctional that both have to be restored to develop a functional occlusion. In that situation some centric stop stability must be maintained until the restorative treatment is done.

Another aspect of the occlusal adjustment and a restorative treatment that must be considered in advance is placement of the margins of restorations. A margin should not involve a centric stop or an end-to-end contact (as in Figure 9–4A,B). With convexity of the axial surface, small areas are often worn at the margins, which tend to open up because of the wear and stresses in working movements, especially with bruxism. Broad, flat surfaces are also contraindicated. A general rule is to place margins outside the zone of contact (between a and b in Figure 9–4C). When esthetics may be a problem because of a margin being placed toward the cervical (slightly beyond a), some adjustment of the maxillary premolar may be possible. The problem of margins opening up in patients with bruxism is especially prominent with feather-edge preparations.

If possible, do not grind on the margins of restorations in the occlusal adjustment. However, a major centric stop should not be sacrificed to avoid the margin. Formation of a new margin may be necessary.

Centric Relation Contacts

One very important point seems to be missed when the mandible is moved into centric relation: the horizontal overlap of the maxillary arch over the mandibular arch increases. Depending on degree of tooth rotation, if any, and the shape of the arch (ovoid, tapering, square), premature contacts occur most often on the lingual inclines of the buccal cusps of the mandibular teeth (Fig. 9–5). These premature contacts involve the distal inclines of the triangular ridges. The more tapering the arch and the greater the distal placement of the mandible, the less will be the horizontal overlap of the maxillary molars and bicuspids and the closer to the cusp tips of the mandibular teeth will be the premature contacts in centric relation.

A very common premature contact in centric relation involves a supporting cusp tip, the distobuccal cusp of the mandibular first molar. There is seldom a problem in deciding where to grind; grinding should be done on the oblique ridge of the maxillary molar.

Because the cusp tip and the distal cusp ridge would be undermined or removed, grinding on the mandibular bicuspid is contraindicated. The cusp tip of the bicuspid is a supporting cusp and the distal cusp ridge is a functional ridge in working.

COMPLETION OF ADJUSTMENT

Completion of Centric Relation Adjustment

The contact vertical dimension at centric relation should be the same as that at centric occlusion at the incisors or at the incisal pin of the articulator. If the incisal pin is set in contact with the incisal table in centric occlusion, the pin will be above

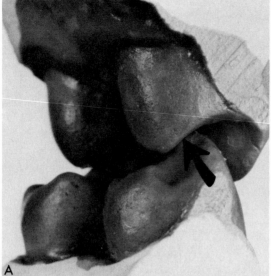

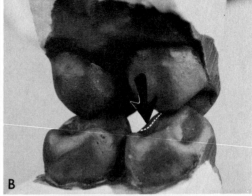

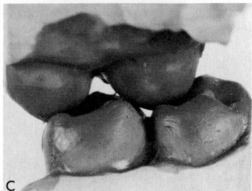

Figure 9–5. Premature contact in centric relation. *A,* premature contact in centric relation; *B,* dotted line indicates area of slide in centric; *C,* centric occlusion position. Adjustment must be done on maxillary premolar and should not involve cusp tip or distal cusp ridge of the mandibular premolar.

the table in centric relation at a height equal to the height of the premature contact. When the premature contact has been eliminated, the incisal pin will contact the table, and the slide in centric will be eliminated.

Completion of Working Side Adjustment

The working side adjustment is completed when it is possible to move the maxillary cast in a lateral and lateral-protrusive direction without interference — that is, a smooth uninterrupted glide from centric outward to an end-to-end relation of buccal cusps, and return to centric. This means from centric occlusion, centric relation, and between centric relation and centric occlusion. Only a small amount of the maxillary teeth should be removed to make multiple contacts. Picking up one or two additional contacts for experience is all that should be done and then only when grinding on anterior teeth would not be required as a result of such grinding, and only when additional

grinding of the balancing side would not result in the elimination of centric stops on the balancing side.

Completion of Balancing Side Adjustment

The balancing side adjustment is considered to be completed on casts when interferences to smooth gliding lateral movements from centric relation and centric occlusion have been eliminated. If necessary, a maxillary lingual cusp centric stop involved in a balancing interference may be removed, but the lingual cusp should not be mutilated. Grinding away or undermining the distal buccal cusp of the mandibular molar or grinding a slot or channel between the distal buccal and distal cusps is contraindicated.

Completion of Protrusive Adjustment

The protrusive adjustment is completed when all interferences to smooth gliding have been removed. All contact guidance should be on the maxillary cuspids and incisors. Grinding of lingual aspects of the maxillary incisors should be limited to very moderated grinding, since the major consideration for grinding in this area is based on an evaluation of the patient. Only rarely is grinding done on lower anterior teeth except in the presence of anterior cross-bite.

PRINCIPLES OF ADJUSTMENT

Supporting Cusps and Centric Stops

Principle. Supporting buccal cusp and cusp ridges of mandibular molar teeth have contact function in both centric and eccentric positions; supporting lingual cusp and cusp ridges of maxillary molars have, or should have, contact only in centric.

Principle. Adjust away from function and centric stops.

Rule. Do not grind on mandibular molar buccal cusp tips or cusp ridges to remove an occlusal interference.

Principle. Supporting buccal cusp and cusp ridges of mandibular premolar teeth have contact function in both centric and eccentric positions; supporting lingual cusp and cusp ridges of maxillary premolars have, or should have, contact only in centric.

Principle. Occlusal forces should be directed (supported) in the long axis of a tooth.

Rule. Do not grind the buccal cusp tip or cusp ridges of the mandibular premolars.

Marginal Ridges

Principle. The occlusal surfaces of approximating marginal ridges are, or may be, the location of centric stops, and the relationship of interproximal contacts, centric stops, and embrasure areas must be maintained to prevent food impaction.

Rule. Do not grind a marginal ridge below the height of the adjacent marginal ridge and do not encroach on the embrasure area.

Unit 9 Exercises

1. When is the centric relation adjustment completed?

   The interferences at centric relation contact (CRC) will be eliminated when: the slide in centric is gone, centric relation equals centric occlusion, freedom of centric has been obtained, contact vertical dimension at centric relation-centric occlusion is attained, or all have been accomplished. (Underline the one most correct answer.)

2. What assumptions must be made in relation to answers for the preceding question?

   The answer would presuppose that: all centric stops have been maintained that existed before the adjustment, the marginal ridges have not been destroyed functionally, the cusp tips and cusp ridges of none of the mandibular buccal cusps have been ground upon, supporting cusp tips were on flat surfaces when possible and not on inclined planes, or all of the above. (Underline the one most correct answer.)

3. When is the working side adjustment completed?

   Working interferences to smooth lateral movements will be eliminated: when there is a cusp guidance, when most of the buccal cusps make contact from centric occlusion outward for at least 2 mm, when a balancing interference (when present) to working cuspid contact has been eliminated, when there is smooth lateral movement with optimal working contacts, or all of foregoing. (Underline the one most correct answer.)

4. When is the balancing side adjustment completed?

   Balancing side interferences will be eliminated: when all contact on the nonfunctional or orbiting side has been eliminated, when all buccal cusps make contact in working on the functioning or working (rotating side), at least there is light or no contact on the balancing side and there are optimal contacts on the working side of the cuspids and lateral incisors, or all of the above. (Underline the one most correct answer.)

5. What key word(s) must be defined in determining the answer to the preceding question?

   _____

   _____

6. Considering the absence of an actual patient and data from a clinical examination, one must view the adjustment of balancing and working on casts as: an estimate, a diagnostic aid, an exercise for beginners, a good guide to the adjustment on the patient, to be done only when indicated, or all of the foregoing. (Underline the one most correct answer.)

7. When will the protrusive adjustment be completed?

   When there are no posterior contacts on any teeth (including the mandibular first premolars) in straight protrusive and slight lateral protrusive, when all guidance is on the maxillary cuspids, when all the incisors and cuspids make contact in straight and slightly lateral protrusive, when there is no in-teference to smooth gliding contact, when there is smooth, gliding contact and the teeth do no move in protrusive movements, or all of the above. (Underline the one most correct answer.)

8. What should be done about supporting cusps contacting inclined planes in "centric"?

In the clinical situation after an occlusal adjustment, there still may be supporting cusps having centric stops on inclined planes. Such a relation-ship: must be changed by further adjustment, might require stabilization by new restorations, is unstable and requires treatment at this time, must be observed until shifting occurs, should be stabilized with an occlusal bit splint, must be treated orthodontically, or all of the foregoing. (Underline the one most correct answer.)

9. What should be done when a supporting cusp makes contact on only one of two approximating marginal ridges of unequal height?

When there are approximating marginal ridges of unequal height as be-tween No. 30 and No. 31 (right mandibular first and second molar) and the supporting cusps make contact with only one of the marginal ridges: the higher marginal ridge should be ground down to the height of the other, the lower should be raised to the height of the highest marginal ridge so that contact may be made on both marginal ridges, the entire occlusion needs restoring, cast data should be correlated with clinical data before any adjusting or restoring is done, this situation is not a problem if no clinical evidence exists to support intervention by adjustment and/or restorations, or none of the above. (Underline the one most correct answer.)

10. In an occlusal adjustment, if there has to be a choice between loss of the centric stop of the distal buccal cusp of the mandibular molar and loss of the centric stop of the mesial lingual cusp of the maxillary first molar because of a balancing interference, which centric stop should be sacrificed?

_____

_____

Unit 9 Test

1. The requirements of an acceptable technique of occlusal adjustment in-clude all the following *except:*

   a. elimination of premature contacts and occlusal interferences
   b. establishment of optimal masticatory effectiveness
   c. providing for stable occlusal relationships
   d. establishment of an efficient pattern of function converging toward centric relation
   e. no exceptions

2. Relative to mandibular supporting cusps and opposing fossae, the cusp is ground:

    a. only when it makes a premature contact in centric and lateral excursions

    b. when it makes a premature contact in centric and not in lateral excursions

    c. when it is "high" in both centric relation and centric occlusion (rarely)

    d. when it is a premature contact in centric relation, centric occlusion and protrusive excursions

    e. none of the above

3. Centric stops:

    a. should never be removed

    b. if required to be removed, this should be done according to the BULL rule

    c. may be required to be removed, but under very specific rules

    d. on inclined planes require occlusal or marginal restorations or both

    e. at centric relation are always superior to those at centric occlusion even after an occlusal adjustment

4. As a guide for an occlusal adjustment, a rule that should be followed is:

    a. maximal functional contact should be maintained around centric

    b. grinding of the lingual axial contours of maxillary teeth should be avoided

    c. avoid grinding the buccal axial contours of mandibular teeth

    d. occlusal interferences in protrusive involving anterior teeth should be adjusted on the lingual surfaces of maxillary teeth

    e. all of the above

5. A premature contact in centric involving a mandibular premolar:

    a. should be ground only after the maxillary premolar has been ground

    b. may be ground before the maxillary premolar if grinding does not involve the cusp tip or ridge

    c. is always ground first when in cross-bite

    d. cannot be ground without creating a step between centric relation and centric occlusion

    e. none of the above

6. Excessive grinding is characterized by:

    a. unnecessary loss of centric stops

    b. loss of functional margin and cusp ridges

    c. a and b

    d. grinding for group function if unnecessary

    e. a, b, and d

7. Excessive grinding on patients can lead to:

    a. pulpitis

    b. dentin sensitivity

    c. occlusal instability

    d. temporomandibular-joint–muscle pain dysfunction

    e. all of the above

8. The first step in the occlusal adjustment on casts is to:

    a. mark balancing interferences and premature contacts
    b. mark centric stops and supporting cusps
    c. adjust working
    d. adjust balancing side interferences
    e. adjust protrusive interferences

9. The rule for adjustment of supporting buccal cusps and cusp ridges of mandibular molar teeth is:

    a. grind away from function
    b. do not grind on mandibular molar buccal cusp tips or cusp ridges
    c. grind toward the interference
    d. adjust to centric relation
    e. none of the above

10. Balancing side adjustment is completed when:

    a. dentin is exposed
    b. balancing side contacts are removed
    c. teeth are no longer mobile
    d. grinding of the balancing side results in smooth gliding movements
    e. none of the above

Unit 10

Waxing Functional Occlusion–1

In waxing the occlusal surfaces of restorations it is necessary to relate the form of the occlusion to the way the teeth come together during mastication, swallowing, and even for parafunction (bruxism). Relating occlusal form to function through a system of waxing and use of an articulator is the major objective of this unit.

The three teeth to be waxed in this unit are all maxillary teeth: the right central incisor, cuspid, and first molar. The occlusion of the incisor is determined by the form of the adjacent incisors and the anterior determinates — that is, the incisal guide is set principally by the contact patterns and facets of wear of the anterior teeth. The occlusion of the cuspid is set by the anterior and posterior determinants, including the absence of balancing contacts and need for working contacts.* The occlusion of the molar is determined principally by posterior determinants, viz., posterior contact patterns, facets of wear, and condylar inclination. The movements of the articulator with the teeth in contact are used to determine cusp height, ridge and groove direction, and the degree of lingual concavity of the maxillary anterior teeth. Thus the determinants of occlusion on the articulator are tooth guidance (including contact patterns and facets of wear), condylar inclination, and articulator movements.

It is recognized that waxing of the occlusal surfaces is only a part of waxing procedure. Margins, gingival contours, proximal contacts, and interproximal morphological features are also important. These aspects will not be considered here.

INTRODUCTION: UNIT OBJECTIVE AND READING

The objective of this unit is to discuss the waxing of three teeth, in which the determinants of occlusion vary because of their type and position. In doing so, several behavioral objectives are desirable.

A. Objectives
1. Be able to give the sequence of steps used in waxing a functional occlusion.
2. Be able to indicate the functions of each part of the occlusal surface to be waxed and how each part is developed in sequence as it comes into function.
3. Be able to wax the occlusal surfaces of the maxillary central incisor, cuspid, and molar, using a wax-added method.
4. Be able to relate what effect the absence of an occlusal adjustment and failure to mount casts in centric relation have on waxing to functional occlusion.
B. Readings* (optional)
Huffman, R. W.: Occlusal morphology (Part 6). *In* Guichet, N. F., Procedures for Occlusal Treatment: A teaching Atlas. Anaheim, Denar Corp., 1968.
Thomas, P. K.: Syllabus on Full Mouth

---

*The need for working side contacts varies with each patient. Group function is not mandatory.

*Videotapes covering the occlusal examination of a patient, analysis of casts, and waxing procedures are available: "Waxing Occlusion in Harmony with Mandibular Movements." Videotapes are produced in U-matic format with audio on track 2. Tapes are also available in Quadruplex, IVC Helical, and E1AJ–1 formats. For further information contact Dr. Major M. Ash, Chairman, Department of Occlusion, School of Dentistry, University of Michigan, Ann Arbor, MI 48109.

Waxing Technique for Rehabilitation. San Diego, Instant Printing Service, 1967.

WAXING TECHNIQUES

Two methods are in general use for waxing restorations outside the mouth: the wax-added and the wax carving techniques. The latter has been called the "smash and carve" method because a bulk of wax is placed on a die and carved after being heated and the articulator closed to the proper contact vertical dimension.

Another variation in the wax carving technique is to generate part of the wax pattern in the mouth and complete the remainder on a die in working casts. In this technique, softened wax is placed in the cavity preparation and the patient is guided through various mandibular excursions with the teeth in contact. This functionally generated wax pattern is completed on the die. This indirect technique is not ideal for waxing of full crowns and for multiple restorations. Direct waxing of completed wax patterns in the mouth is not widely used.

Several wax-added, add-on, or wax-to-wax techniques have been developed to enable step-by-step control of waxing so that cusps, fossae, and ridges can be formed in relation to excursions of the articulator. In the technique presented here, one or two aspects of the occlusion can be developed at a time rather than all aspects of the occlusion having to be considered at once. Supporting cusps can be accurately placed and occlusal stability enhanced. It is especially useful for diagnostic waxing.

In the development of the waxed restoration an objective is to have some parts of occlusal surfaces make contact and other surfaces to be free of contact in centric occlusion and in various excursions. Areas that should contact are developed by adding small amounts of wax until contact is established. The areas that will be free of contact are developed to be short of contact to avoid interference with function.

The wax-added technique described here can be used for single as well as multiple restorations or a full mouth rehabilitation, and is essentially a technique to meet the requirements of the concept of freedom in centric. The technique is appropriate for development of a cusp-to-fossa and cusp-to-marginal ridge occlusion, which is seen most often in the natural dentition and involves a one-tooth to two-teeth arrangement. However, it can be used with any arrangement of teeth.

MOUNTING OF CASTS

This may be accomplished by (1) using a patient's casts mounted in centric relation on an articulator, (2) using a set of standard* casts mounted in simulated centric relation, or (3) mounting the casts in centric occlusion. Method 2 will be used here, but waxing will be done only in and from centric occlusion.

Note: For this unit the casts should not reflect an occlusal adjustment either in the patient or on the casts. One of the objectives of this unit is to demonstrate the potential effect of occlusal interferences in centric relation on waxing procedures.

EQUIPMENT AND MATERIALS

Casts

The casts shown in this unit are from the same subject (Fig. 10–1) as those seen in Units 6, 7, and 9. However, any set of similar casts may be used provided that an occlusal adjustment has not been done on the patient from whom the casts were derived. Ordinarily an occlusal adjustment should have been done, but to demonstrate the relationship to waxing procedures an adjustment is not done.

Waxing Instruments

There are a number of suitable waxing instruments that may be used. For example, the P. K. Thomas No. 1 is excellent for adding drops of wax, the No. 2 for carving

---

*Casts made from the same mould so that it is possible to present the same occlusion to a large number of individuals. The casts are made of stone poured in moulds. The moulds can be made of plastic material in any dental laboratory or purchased from Viade Products, Inc., Camarillo, CA 93010. Standard casts may be purchased from Columbia Dentoform, New York, NY 10010.

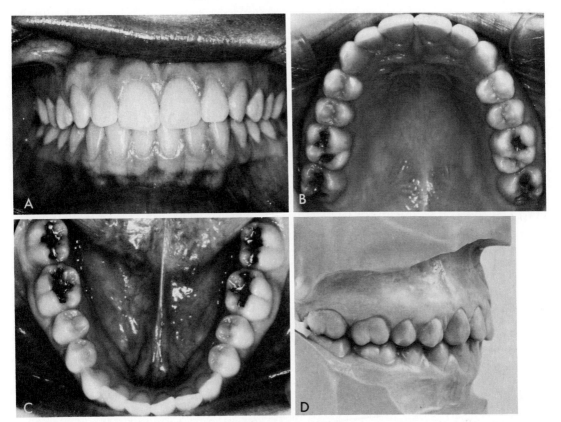

Figure 10-1. *Subject and cast.* The examination of this subject was reviewed in Unit 6. *A,B,C*, clinical views of occlusion; *D*, casts showing right side, which is to be the side of functional waxing.

grooves, and the No. 3 for carving axial and proximal surfaces.*

Waxes

Inlay waxes of various colors and hardness are useful. Different colored waxes† can facilitate waxing different parts but are not essential. The room temperature is a significant factor in the degree of hardness and flow of wax. Soft waxes may be of little value in a warm room. Hard waxes may be so brittle at normal or cool room temperatures that cusps and ridges may break rather easily.

Zinc stearate is very useful for wax lubrication and to determine points of occlusal contact. In this respect a double-ended *plate brush* can be used: the soft end for

applying the zinc stearate and the stiff end to remove wax chips.

28 gauge green sheet wax is used to determine the amount of occlusal reduction that is required.

Removal of Cast Material

Instruments such as a *knife* and/or No. 701 bur and handpiece are necessary to reduce occlusal surface before replacement of anatomical surfaces with wax.

Occlusal Marking Materials

A number of articulating papers are available to detect occlusal contacts. Generally very thin *articulating paper* and *typewriter ribbon* are the most effective. Use of two different colors is suggested to mark different jaw positions. Both paper and ribbon must be freshly made (or

---

*American Dental Mfg. Co., Missoula, MO 59801.

†Delar Rainbow Color-Coded Waxes, Almore International Inc., Portland, OR 97225.

sealed) and prevented from drying in the air in order to be effective.

Thin cellophane silver *shim stock** is recommended for testing the absence of occlusal contacts.

GOALS FOR WAXING

Centric stops should be located in stable areas. Supporting cusp contacts should be stable. Posterior contacts should be between cusp tips and flat occlusal stops in fossae (Fig. 10–2). Light contact on incisors is desirable.

The supporting cusp tips of posterior teeth should be located in the central groove area to allow protrusive movement without posterior contacts. Triangular ridges often interfere with protrusive movement unless care is taken in the waxing.

Contact of the incisors in protrusive should be related to other anterior contacts. Canine contacts may take precedence over the central and lateral incisors in lateral protrusive movement but should not prevent edge-to-edge contact of the incisors in straight protrusive.

The only parts making contact in centric should be the tips of the supporting cusps and centric stops. The posterior supporting cusps should not make contact on the balancing side.

*Artus Corp., Englewood, NJ 07631.

The nonsupporting cusps should be smaller, shorter, and nearer the outer edges of the occlusal surfaces than the supporting cusps. This is done to prevent contact of these cusps in centric occlusion.

Height of the nonsupporting cusps should be consistent with that of the adjacent teeth, not only for the maxillary posterior teeth but also for the maxillary incisors. The lingual cusps of the mandibular posterior teeth must provide protection against tongue biting.

The vertical and horizontal overlap of the posterior maxillary teeth must be consistent with the width of the occlusal surfaces, must provide working contact when appropriate, and must prevent cheek biting.

Marginal ridges of waxed restorations should be the same height as those of adjacent teeth. Ridges and grooves should follow the same direction as mandibular movements.

PREPARATION FOR WAXING

The articulator will be set in two positions in this unit: (1) centric occlusion of the casts for the initial waxing and (2) centric relation at the completion of waxing for analysis of the influence of not doing an occlusal adjustment and not waxing to function in centric relation as well as centric occlusion.

*Note: To prevent wear of the stone, the occlusal surfaces of the casts should be painted with a protective coating.**

Mounting of Casts

Check to see that the articulator is zeroed.

If using an ear piece face bow, set the condylar inclination to 70. Mount the maxillary cast using the face bow and bite plane (fork). Set the inclination of the occlusal plane with the molar end of casts inclined down 10° to 15°. The incisal edge of the maxillary incisors should be *at* or *between* the scribe lines on the straight incisal pin.

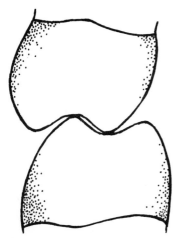

Figure 10–2. *Goals of waxing.* A principal goal is to have supporting cusps make contact with flat planes.

*W/G 1-in-3, Sealer, Hardner, Spacer. Williams Dental Instruments, 520 Wildwood, Park Forest, IL 60466.

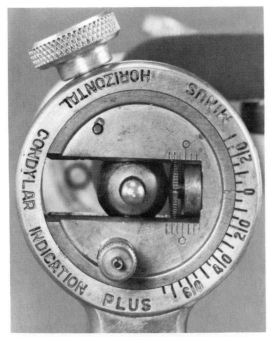

Figure 10–3. *Simulated centric relation mounting.* Condylar stops are set back distance desired for slide in centric and cast mounted in centric occlusion.

Set the condylar stop counterclockwise to 1 mm beyond zero (Fig. 10–3). If the articulator does not have a PR adjustment, use a 0.20 in brass or plastic shim.

Set the condylar inclination to 25 and lateral inclination to 15. *Because the condylar shaft is now not centered in the condylar guidance, the condylar guidance cannot be moved without causing disclusion of centric stops in centric occlusion.*

Mount the mandibular cast in centric occlusion using quick-setting impression plaster. Set the incisal guide table and customize if necessary to maximize tooth guidance (See Unit 3).

Identification of Occlusal Surfaces

Inasmuch as each part of the occlusal surfaces of a tooth is developed in wax according to its function, these parts should be identified. On the casts mounted on the articulator, identify the centric stops, supporting cusps and nonsupporting cusps on the *left* mandibular teeth. Mark with pencil lines on the buccal surfaces of the supporting cusps of the mandibular teeth.

Identify the cusp ridges, marginal ridges, triangular ridges, and major grooves on the left side. Indicate the position of the buccal and lingual grooves with a pencil.

Identify the centric stops, supporting cusps and nonsupporting cusps on the left maxillary teeth. Mark with a pencil.

Identify and mark the path of the supporting cusps of working and balancing sides and for protrusive movement.

Preparation of Teeth

The maxillary *right* central incisor, right cuspid, and right maxillary first molar are prepared by removing 2 to 3 mm of stone from the occlusal surfaces (Fig. 10–4). Enough of the lingual surface and incisal edge of the maxillary right central incisor is removed to allow adequate wax to be added so that contact of the stone does not occur in protrusive and lateral protrusive movements.

As the stone is removed, the articulator member should be moved in various excursions to assure clearance in all possible occlusal contact relations. The reduced surface should follow the original tooth form.

When the surface appears to have been sufficiently removed, place five thicknesses of 28 gauge green wax on the reduced surfaces and move the articulator member through various excursions to detect contacts. If contacts are present, reduce the surface at the point of contact.

Wax Handling

Proper waxing can be accomplished only if the flow of wax is controlled through proper heating of the waxing instruments. If the wax is too cold, it will not flow. If it is too hot, it will flow out of control. The control of heat is best accomplished by proper transfer of heat to the instrument and from the instrument to the wax.

The waxing instrument should be heated with the blue tip part of the flame (reducing part). The instrument is passed through the flame so that the blue tip of the flame concentrates the heat about one half inch from the tip of the blade of the instrument (Fig. 10–5). In order to see the tip of the instrument and flame, use of a black

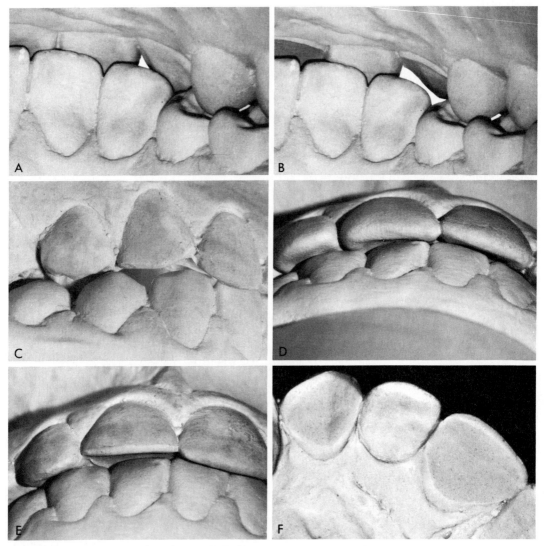

Figure 10–4. *Preparation of casts. A, B, C,* preparation of cuspid; *D, E, F,* preparation of incisor.

Illustration continued on opposite page

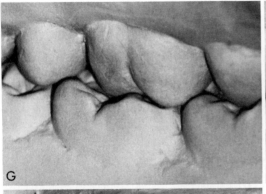
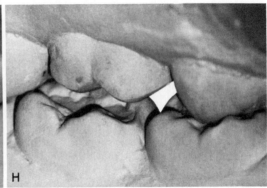
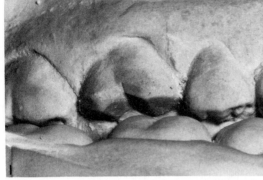

Figure 10–4. *Continued. G, H, I,* preparation of molar.

background is helpful. Blackened metal or a bunsen burner shield* can be used.

As an exercise, practice developing wax cones on a flat surface of plaster or stone. First spread a layer of ivory-colored wax over the surface. The PKT No. 1 or other suitable instrument is passed through the flame, keeping the tip away from the flame so that the wax will flow toward the tip rather than toward the handle (Fig. 10–5A). Make contact with the wax to be used at the place on the blade that has been heated (Fig. 10–5B). A drop of molten wax should adhere toward the tip of the instrument's blade (Fig. 10–5C). If necessary, carry the blade back through the flame again but away from the wax. Practice is necessary to develop the proper timing to control the heat. A further appreciation for the proper amount of heat can be obtained by forming cones on the thumbnail. This exercise should not be attempted until some facility for controlling wax has been developed.

The waxed tip of the PKT No. 1 is placed in contact with the waxed plaster or stone.

If heated correctly the wax should flow down the instrument to form a mound. In a circular movement remove the tip slowly from contact with the stone and allow the wax to cool and solidify just as the tip of the blade is removed from the cone of wax. The wax is added incrementally in this way until a cone of the correct height is formed. In this instance, develop cones that are 3 mm in height 5 to 6 mm apart. When you master the art of forming cones, practice connecting the cones with ridges to simulate cusp ridges. Then practice making cones and triangular ridges.

Outline of Steps in Waxing (Fig. 10–6)

Step 1. Locate and mark centric stops on prepared and opposing teeth.
Step 2. Develop supporting cusps (Fig. 10–6A).
Step 3. Develop centric stops for the opposing supporting cusps (Fig. 10–6B).
Step 4. Develop the nonsupporting cusps (Fig. 10–6C).
Step 5. Develop the cusp ridges, marginal ridges, and the axial contours (Fig. 10–6D).

*Bunsen Burner Shield, Almore International, Portland, OR 97227.

Text continued on page 161

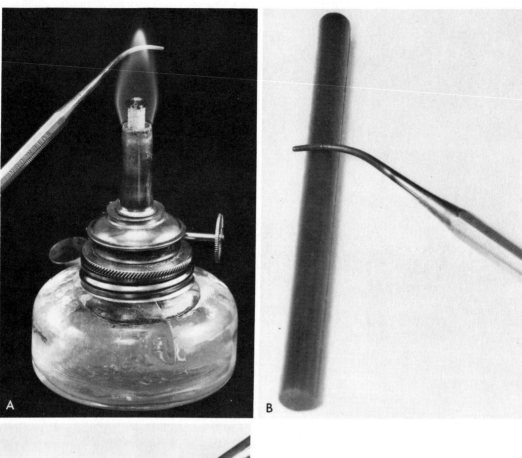

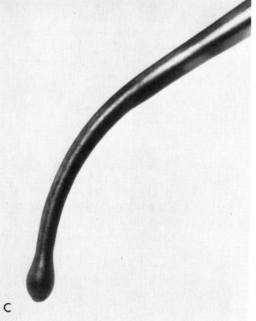

Figure 10–5. *Wax handling. A,* position of waxing instrument in flame; *B,* picking up wax; *C,* drop of molten wax on tip of instrument. (See text.)

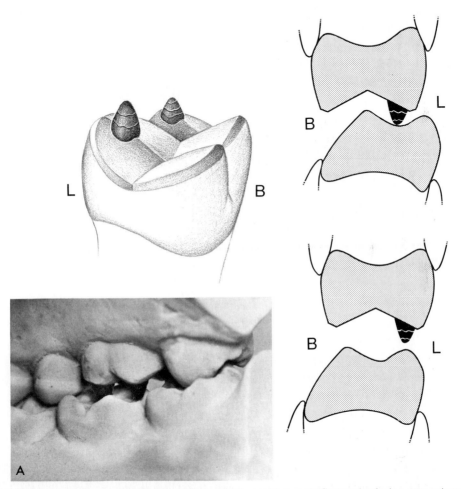

Figure 10–6A. *Develop supporting cusps. Upper Left,* maxillary right first molar facing upward on opened upper member of articulator. The cusp cones for the lingual cusps have been developed in wax. B, buccal; L, lingual. *Lower left,* waxed cones occluding on centric stops of lower first molar. *Upper right,* supporting cusp tip in contact with centric stop, which was marked in step 1 on the mandibular first molar. *Lower right,* lateral movements such as right working and protrusive should be made to ensure that waxed cusps do not clash.

Illustration continued on following page

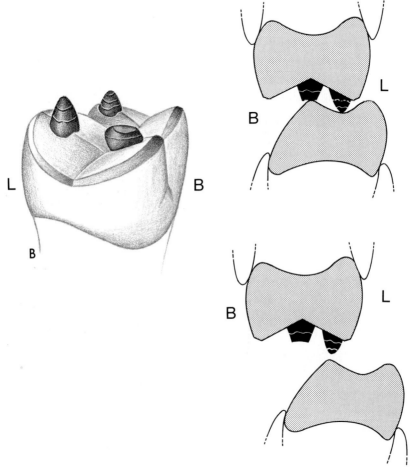

Figure 10–6B. *Develop centric stops. Left,* centric stop for distal buccal cusp of mandibular right first molar is developed as shown in the central fossa area of the maxillary first molar. *Upper right,* height of centric stop is established in centric occlusion. *Lower right,* curvature of centric is established in eccentric movements and protrusive excursions.

Illustration continued on opposite page

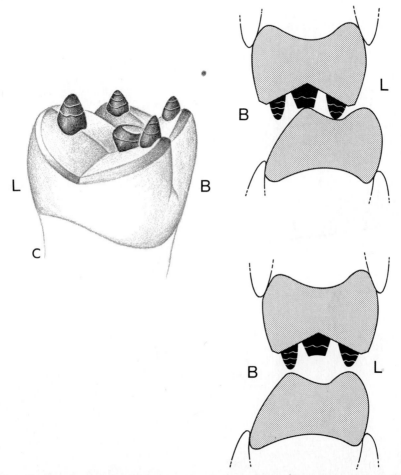

Figure 10–6C. *Develop nonsupporting cusps. Left,* buccal nonsupporting cusps developed. *Upper right,* buccal cusps height related to height of other posterior buccal cusps on the right side and to the amount of horizontal overlap required. *Lower right,* height of cusp should be related to functional movements.

Illustration continued on following page

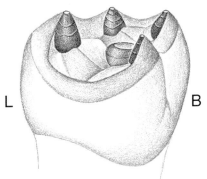

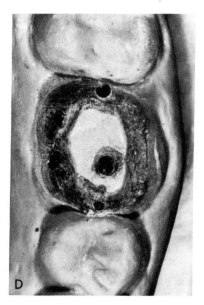

Figure 10–6D. Develop cusp ridges, marginal ridges and axial contours. *Upper,* cusp ridges are formed in relation to lateral and protrusive movements. There should be no contact of distal cusp ridge of the distal buccal cusp in protrusive. Contact of buccal cusp ridges in lateral does not occur in complete cuspid disclusion but may occur in some instances if group function is present. There should be no contact of lingual cusp ridges in centric (CR or CO) or in lateral movements. There should be no contact of buccal cusp ridges in centric (CR or CO). Marginal ridges should make contact only in centric (CR or CO) as centric stops. Axial contours should not make contact in any position or movement. *Lower,* waxed cusp ridges, marginal ridges, and axial contours.

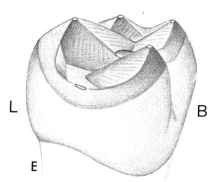

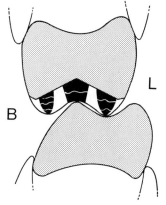

Figure 10–6E. Develop triangular ridges. *Left,* triangular ridges are formed so that no contact occurs in centric relation or centric occlusion and in protrusive or balancing movements. Contacts in working are related to group function or cuspid disclusion or both. *Right,* triangular ridges and axial surfaces are free of contact in centric.

Illustration continued on opposite page

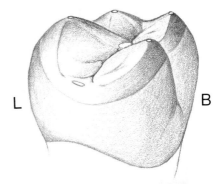

L   B

Figure 10–6F. Completion of waxing. *Upper and lower,* the wax is smoothed and then dusted with zinc stearate to demonstrate presence of centric stops on supporting cusps (L), in central fossa, and on the mesial and distal marginal ridges. There are no other contacts in centric. The wax cone tips are still visible on the buccal (B) nonsupporting cusps. *Lower,* the only contact marks allowed in lateral and protrusive movements are those involving the lingual aspects of the buccal cusps in working provided such function is indicated. None are allowed in protrusive.

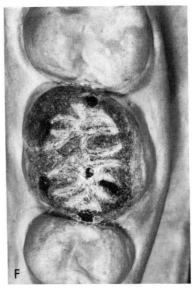

Step 6. Develop triangular ridges and grooves (Fig. 10–6E) and complete waxing (Fig. 10–6F).

WAXING FOR FUNCTION

The principles to be described are suitable for most occlusal relations; however, the illustrations relate to a standard or normal occlusion with minor variations. The paths for cusp movements are shown in Figure 10–7. A knowledge of the paths of supporting cusps aids in deciding where to guide the articulator during the waxing procedure.

Step 1. *Locate Centric Stops on the Opposing (Existing) Occlusion*

Centric stops are located near "escapeways" (grooves between cusps) that permit the supporting cusp to function without clashing with other cusps and without interferences from other parts of the tooth surface.

Note: Not all fossae are usable for centric stops because of the movements of the supporting cusps; a maxillary supporting cusp placed in the mandibular mesial fossae would, in a balancing movement, clash with the cusps of the mandibular teeth (Fig. 10–8).

Locate and mark centric stops for the proposed supporting cusps on the opposing occlusal surfaces of the casts. The occlusal relationships that can be considered to enhance occlusal stability include: (1) a supporting cusp tip contacting a flat area in a fossa, (2) a supporting cusp with a flat tip contacting a marginal ridge, (3) a supporting cusp with a flat tip contacting two marginal ridges (cusp does not extend into embrasure), and (4) a supporting cusp tip contacting a flat area in a distal fossa (Fig. 10–9).

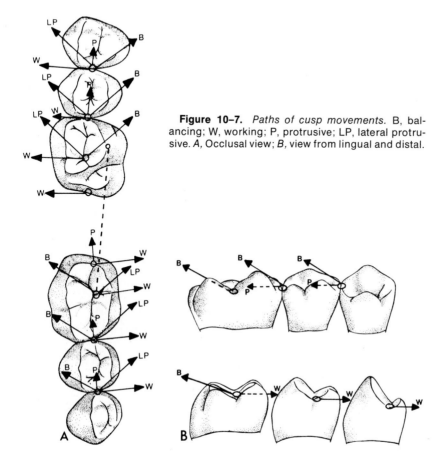

Figure 10–7. *Paths of cusp movements.* B, balancing; W, working; P, protrusive; LP, lateral protrusive. *A,* Occlusal view; *B,* view from lingual and distal.

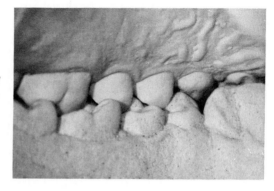

Figure 10–8. *Relationship of cusps to fossa and potential for clashing of cusps during movement.* (See text.)

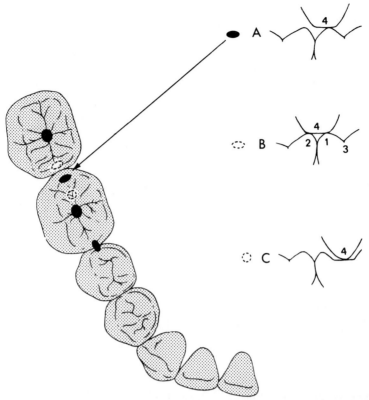

Figure 10–9. *Waxing–Step 1.* Locating centric stops. 1, distal marginal ridge of mandibular first molar (No. 30); 2, mesial marginal ridge of mandibular second molar (No. 3); 3, distal fossa of No. 30; 4, distal lingual cusps of No. 3.

Not all fossae are usable for centric stops because of the movements of the supporting cusps; that is, a maxillary supporting cusp placed in the mandibular mesial fossae would, in a balancing movement, clash with the cusps of the mandibular teeth.

Cusps that occlude on only one marginal ridge as in A, Figure 10–9, may allow the distal molar to drift distally. For example, the distal lingual cusp of the maxillary right first molar should occlude where necessary for occlusal stability on the distal marginal ridge of the mandibular right first molar and on the mesial marginal ridge of the mandibular right second molar.

As an exercise, draw on Figure 10–9 the position of centric stops and movement paths made by supporting cusps of the right mandibular incisor, cuspid, and molar.

Step 2. *Develop Supporting Cusp Tips*

The *supporting cusps* are the buccal cusps of the mandibular premolars and molars, the lingual cusps of the maxillary premolars and molars, and the incisal edges of the mandibular anterior teeth.

Using the No. 1 waxing instrument, add wax to develop the cusp cones from the prepared tooth toward the marked opposing centric stops. Add small amounts of wax until the top of the cusp contacts the centric occlusion stop (Figs. 10–10 and 10–11). Using the soft end of the plate brush, dust zinc stearate powder onto the freshly added part. Zinc stearate acts as a lubricant and also indicates contacts. The surface is dulled by the zinc stearate. Contacts with opposing surface make shiny areas. The stiff bristle end of the plate brush is used to remove excess zinc stearate and wax chips that tend to accumulate on the waxed surfaces. When contact is established, move the supporting cusp in the articulator movements to determine its relationship with the existing parts of the opposing occlusion.

Throughout the entire waxing procedure the articulator movements are made with each wax addition to determine (1) if

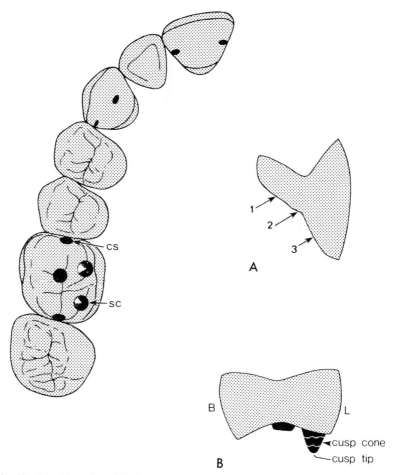

Figure 10–10. *Waxing–Steps 2 and 3.* Step 2: Development of supporting cusp tips (sc); Step 3: Development of centric stops (cs) for the opposing supporting cusps. B, buccal; L, lingual; 1, 2, 3, potential position for centric stops.

parts are needed for contact or guidance and (2) if the shape of the part is affected by the interaction of the opposing tooth elements. If the answer to both these questions is no, the part is formed according to ideal tooth morphology.

Functional Criteria. Reposition the waxed cusp as needed to establish three functional criteria from centric occlusion: protrusive movement, working movement, and balancing movement.

1. Protrusive movement–no posterior tooth contacts. Position the supporting cusp cones buccally or lingually until they are in the center of the opposing tooth. This also places the forces more along the long axis of the tooth. The opposing central groove provides space for supporting cusps to move into protrusive excursions (Fig. 10–7). The anterior teeth should contact in protrusive.

2. Working movement–either the canine alone or several teeth on the working side may provide working contacts. Position the cusp cones mesial or distal to an embrasure or a fossa and near grooves or escapeways depending on whether contact or clearance is required (Figs. 10–10 and 10–11A,B).

3. Balancing movement–no posterior tooth should contact on the balancing side. Tooth contacts and guidances on the working side keep the cusps from contacting on the balancing side.

Unworn supporting cusp tips are relatively pointed but are rounder, broader, and longer than nonsupporting cusps. Excessively flattened cusps require wider fossae and grooves. Supporting cusp tips are the highest elevations on the occlusal surface; therefore, they will clash in function if they are not developed in proper harmony with mandibular movements.

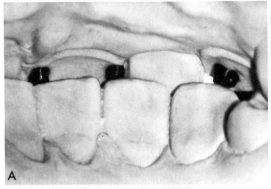
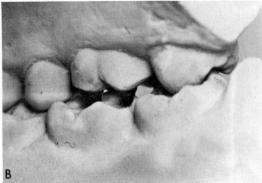
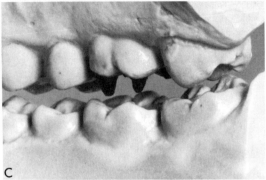

Figure 10–11. *Waxing to function.* Development of supporting cusp tips on incisor and cuspid (*A*) and on the molar (*B*); evaluation of cusp tips for clearance in working for first molar (*C*). Centric stops for incisor may be developed on marginal ridges in step 5.

The height of a cusp is related to condylar and incisal determinants and to depth and direction of the grooves (passageways).

The supporting cusp tips and their opposing centric stop are the *only* parts that need to contact when the teeth are closed into centric.

Develop each part on the three prepared teeth before going to the next step.

Step 3. *Develop Centric Stops for the Opposing Supporting Cusps*

Mark the tips of the opposing supporting cusps with a pencil. Add small amounts of the wax to the potential centric stop area until it contacts the supporting cusp in centric occlusion. Warm the wax again, then move the supporting cusp in the mandibular movements. Establish the functional criteria listed in Step 2. Cusp to fossa stops and cusp to marginal ridge stops will be developed in this step (Fig. 10–10).

Centric stops on anterior teeth may be located at the cingulum or marginal ridges as in A shown in Figure 10–10. *If the anterior teeth are not in near contact,* do not try to establish contact with the teeth

being waxed. Use the contours of the adjacent teeth to determine the lingual surface contour heights of the waxed teeth.

The amount of overjet (horizontal overlap) and overbite (vertical overlap) and the shape of the lingual concavity of maxillary anterior teeth affect the cusp height and fossa depth of the posterior teeth.

Step 4. *Develop the Nonsupporting Cusp Tips*

Nonsupporting cusps are the lingual cusps of the mandibular posterior teeth, the buccal cusps of the maxillary posterior teeth, and the incisal edges of the maxillary anterior teeth. Nonsupporting cusps are smaller, shorter, and nearer to outer edges of the occlusal surface in comparison to the supporting cusps. This difference in position and cusp height accounts for a necessary overjet on posterior teeth.

Add wax to develop the nonsupporting cusps toward the opposing occlusal surfaces. These cusps do not contact opposing surfaces in centric. The lengths of these cusps are determined by the length of the nonsupporting cusps on the adjacent teeth (the depth of the opposing grooves) and

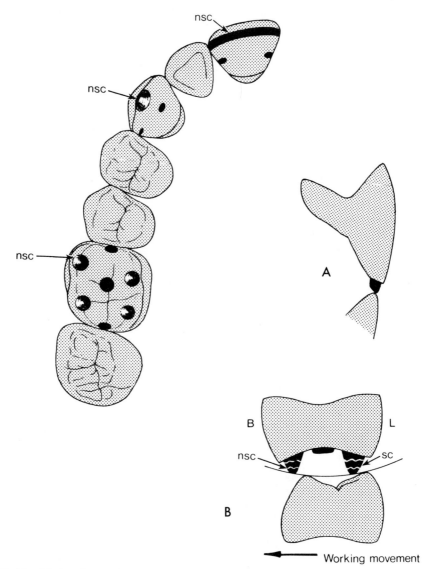

Figure 10–12. *Waxing–Step 4.* Development of nonsupporting cusp tips (nsc): *A,* incisal edge in protrusive; *B,* relationship of supporting (SC) and nonsupporting cusps in working movement. Curved line represents curve of Wilson.

the parameters of movement of the supporting cusps as in A and B, Figure 10–12.

Position the nonsupporting cusps so that they meet the functional criteria listed in Step 2. Contacts between supporting cusps (mandibular posterior) and nonsupporting cusps (maxillary posterior and anterior teeth) can provide tooth guidance for lateral movements as in B, Figure 10–12. Lateral contacts in working may be established on the buccal cusps only.

Step 5. Develop the Cusp Ridges, Marginal Ridges, and the Axial (Cavo-Surface) Contours

The *cusp ridges* or *marginal ridges* or both extend from cusp tip to cusp tip around the circumference of the occlusal surfaces of the posterior teeth and the lingual surfaces of the anterior teeth. These ridges delineate the occlusal and axial surface. On the posterior teeth, these are termed mesial and distal cusp ridges and mesial and distal marginal ridges (Fig. 10–13).

Axial contours extend from the cusp ridges and marginal ridges toward the gingiva. The axial contours are the mesial, distal, buccal (or labial), and lingual shape of the coronal part of a tooth as in B, Figure 10–13.

Add wax to develop the marginal ridges. Portions of the ridges form part of the boundaries of a fossa. Do not form the marginal ridges too close to the supporting cusps or so high as to interfere with the movements of the supporting cusps.

Portions of the marginal ridges can form centric stops — that is, the distal marginal ridges of the mandibular first and second

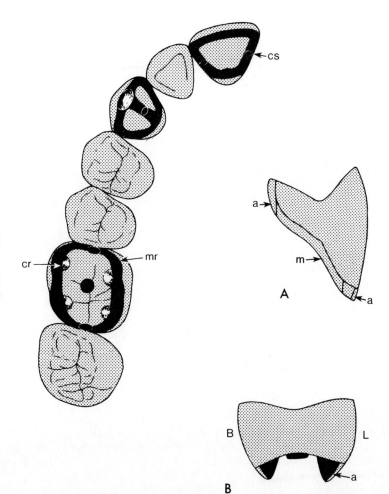

Figure 10–13. *Waxing–Step 5.* Development of cusp ridges (cr) and marginal ridges (mr) and axial (cavosurface) contours (a). Centric stops (cs) may be developed on marginal ridges in this step rather than step 2.

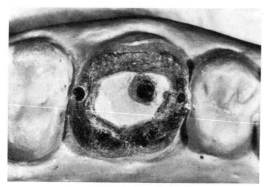

Figure 10–14. *Waxing marginal ridges.* Use of zinc stearate to aid in the development of centric stops on marginal ridges.

molars can provide centric stops for the distal lingual supporting cusps of maxillary first and second molars (Fig. 10–14).

Portions of the cusp ridges can provide guiding inclines in working movements. Check for contact and clearances in all movements according to the functional criteria listed in Step 2.

Add wax to form the axial contours. The shape of the carved axial contour blends with the curvatures of the remaining tooth structure. The axial surface is designed to keep the gingival tissues healthy. Axial surfaces can be overcontoured to produce interferences with the opposing occlusion. Check the axial contours in all mandibular movements. Carving of the axial contours can be done with a No. 4 waxing instrument.

In waxing these areas it is easier (again) to add a segment of wax. Just before the wax hardens completely add zinc stearate, which acts as a lubricant and marks contacts. Bring the newly waxed part into contact and go through the articulator movements. Add wax until the desired form is established. Those areas added that are not needed in contact build into near contact.

Step 6. *Develop Triangular Ridges and Grooves*

Triangular ridges extend from a cusp tip to the central developmental groove (Fig. 10–15). This part is narrow at the cusp tip and wider at the base, where it contacts the opposite triangular ridge — thus it is triangular in shape. The central developmental groove separates two joining triangular ridges and provides space for sup-

porting cusps in protrusive movements. The height of a triangular ridge is determined by the anterior and posterior determinants in protrusive and lateral protrusive movements. The mesial and distal borders are formed by the supplemental grooves or depressions. Triangular ridges together with the marginal ridges form the boundaries of a fossa containing a centric stop.

Triangular ridges are rounded surfaces. In tooth development the parts of the teeth are developed in lobes; therefore, all surfaces are curved. Wax added in drops to develop the parts of the tooth will be curved. Carving the wax and wearing or grinding of a tooth surface create flattened surfaces or areas.

Add wax to develop the triangular ridges. *Do not* alter the height or position of the cusp tips. *Do not* form the ridges too close to the centric stops. The angles of the ridges and the grooves are directed by the movements of the supporting cusps as determined by the anterior and posterior guidance. Check each wax addition in forming the angles of ridges and the angles of the grooves with the movements to prevent the formation of interferences.

Add a small amount of wax to form the remaining occlusal surfaces. Develop the grooves and carvings so that the occlusal surfaces (or lingual surface on anterior) resemble "normal" teeth. The opposite side of the same arch may also be used as a reference. Areas of the occlusal surface that have become flattened from contacts during movements and from carving can be and should be rounded again. Heat the small tip of the No. 1 waxing instrument and remelt these flattened surfaces. Upon cooling, the surface will be round again. *Be sure* to add zinc stearate to this remelted area and evaluate during mandibular movements.

Developmental grooves are formed between two cusp lobes and provide major passageways for the supporting cusps from centric positions to lateral positions (Fig. 10–15). Therefore, the angles of the grooves must be in relationship to the supporting cusps in function. Make sure they are wide enough and deep enough to provide clearances for the cusp tips. Use the waxing instrument No. 3 to sharpen the groove.

Supplemental grooves are small grooves on either side of the triangular ridges di-

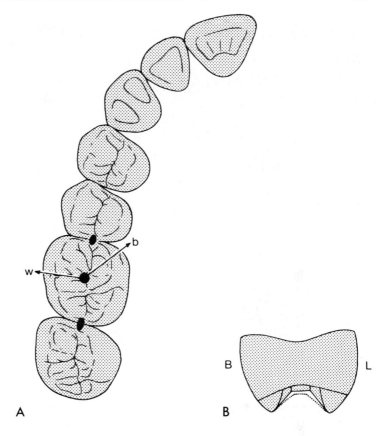

Figure 10–15. *Waxing–Step 6.* Development of triangular ridges and grooves.

viding the occluding surfaces into a series of ridges that break up potential flat surfaces. These grooves minimize the total contact area of the occluding parts and also provide voids and wider grooves for better passageways. Chewing efficiency is related to areas of near contact as well as areas of contact.

OCCLUSAL ANALYSIS (FROM CENTRIC OCCLUSION)

The waxed occlusal surfaces should be analyzed in protrusive, working, and balancing movements. The incisal pin is raised so that the teeth make contact and provide guidance. The waxed surfaces are inspected for contact in working, balancing, and protrusive (Fig. 10–16A,B,C).

Protrusive

Dust the waxed surfaces with zinc stearate. Move the supporting cusps in protrusive and observe the contacts or interferences or both on the waxed occlusion. If necessary, remove wax from the waxed occlusion until the natural teeth and the waxed occlusion contact equally. The anterior teeth provide the guidance for the protrusive movement. The posterior teeth parts should not contact in the protrusive movement.

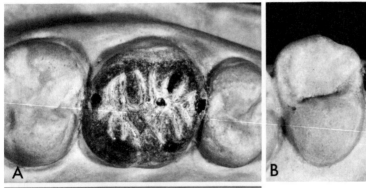
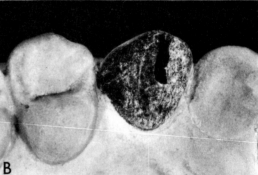
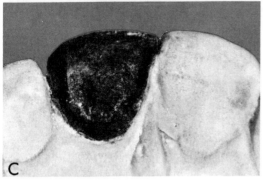

Figure 10–16. Occlusal analysis. Waxed surfaces dusted with zinc stearate and maxillary cast moved into lateral and protrusive positions. *A*, centric stops on molar and light working contact on mesial buccal cusp. *B*, cuspid working contact. *C*, incisor contact in protrusive. No balancing or protrusive contacts are present on molar.

1. *Waxed occlusion*
   a. List the tooth parts (marginal ridge, triangular ridge, and so forth) of the waxed occluding surfaces that have caused interferences (areas where wax was removed) and those parts that have provided guidance (wax just contacted).

GUIDANCE	INTERFERENCES
Central incisor_____	_____
_____	_____
Canine _____	_____
_____	_____
Molar_____	_____
_____	_____

   b. What could be anticipated in waxing occluding surfaces to prevent protrusive interferences?

   _____

   _____

2. After the wax has been analyzed and the natural teeth are in contact, analyze the natural teeth contacts in protrusive. Use red tape (Madame Butterfly) to mark contacts. List the teeth and the parts of the occluding natural teeth that are protrusive interferences.

_____

_____

_____

3. List the tooth contacts that provide guidance in protrusive.

_____

_____

_____

Working and Balancing Movements

Observe the working and balancing side occlusion together for a right and a left lateral articulator movement. Add zinc stearate to the waxed occlusion before movements are made. Make the observations listed below for a right lateral and then a left lateral movement.

1. *Right lateral movement*
   The teeth on the side of the rotating condyle (working side) are in a functioning relationship (buccal cusp to buccal cusp). The teeth on the side of the translating condyle (balancing side) should not be functioning, but idling without contact. The lingual cusps of the maxillary posterior teeth move toward the buccal cusps of the mandibular posterior teeth.
   a. Waxed occlusion (in working): List the parts of the occluding surfaces that cause interferences and those used as guidance.

GUIDANCE	INTERFERENCES
Central incisor_____	_____
_____	_____
Canine _____	_____
_____	_____
Molar _____	_____

   b. What could be anticipated in the waxing occlusion to prevent working interferences?
   c. Analyze the natural teeth in balancing contacts with red tape. List the teeth and tooth surfaces causing balancing interferences.

_____

_____

_____

2. *Left lateral movement*
a. Waxed occlusion (in balancing): List the parts of the waxed occluding surfaces that cause interferences in balancing movements.

Central incisor_____

_____

Canine _____

_____

Molar _____

_____

b. What could be anticipated in waxing occluding surfaces to prevent balancing interferences?

_____

_____

c. Analyze with red tape the natural teeth in working movement. List the teeth and tooth parts of the natural teeth interferences in working movement.

_____

_____

OCCLUSAL ANALYSIS (FROM CENTRIC RELATION)

At the completion of the waxing as well as during waxing of the occlusal surfaces of restorations, the waxing should be related to excursive movements from centric occlusion and centric relation. However, in this exercise the waxing was carried out only from centric occlusion and not centric relation in order to demonstrate the effect of movement into and away from centric relation. Therefore, at this time the articulator is adjusted to allow the casts to be positioned in centric relation. This adjustment allows the effects of centric relation position on the waxings and on the unwaxed teeth to be visualized. Keep in mind that centric relation is a border position (sagittal place) and may be reached at times in function and parafunction.

Adjustment of the Articulator

1. Increase the vertical dimension 3 to 4 mm by use of the incisal pin. This procedure is temporary so as to protect the wax and stone before unintentional heavy contact is made in centric relation.
2. Reset the condylar stop to zero. The casts are now in the simulated centric relation.

Initial Centric Relation Contacts

1. After the adjustment of the PR component, lock the condylar elements in the simulated centric relation position by securing the centric lock thumb-screw.
2. Raise the incisal pin to allow light contact on waxings.
3. Using the blue articulating paper, mark the premature contacts in centric relation. Indicate their location (tooth and tooth part).

   Maxilla _____

   _____

   _____

   Mandible _____

   _____

4. Indicate those involving the waxed teeth (if any).

   _____

   _____

   _____

5. Measure the amount of opening (OP) between the teeth in the area of the central incisors and canines (Fig. 10–17).

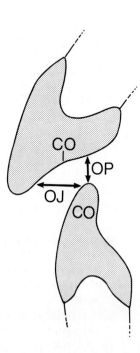

Figure 10–17. Horizontal overlap (OJ) and opening (OP) with condylar elements and stops set at zero (casts in centric relation position).

Central incisors_____

Canines _____

6. Measure the amount of overjet (OJ) in the area of the central incisors and canines.

Central incisors_____

Canines _____

Centric Relation–Centric Occlusion

The center portion of Figure 10–18 is an enlarged view of the area around centric (Posselt's diagram). When there is a premature contact in centric relation closure, any supporting cusp tip in the mandibular arch will be posterior and inferior to its position in centric occlusion. On initial contact in centric relation the mandible is deflected upward and forward and produces a slide from centric relation to centric occlusion. In the sagittal plane the slide in centric has a vertical (m in Figure 10–18) component as well as a horizontal component (1). With the premature contact removed and all interferences to a smooth gliding movement from centric relation to centric occlusion removed, there is then present "freedom in centric." When there is freedom in centric a supporting cusp can freely move from centric relation to centric occlusion without interference.

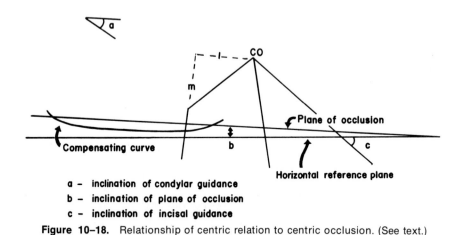

a – inclination of condylar guidance
b – inclination of plane of occlusion
c – inclination of incisal guidance

Figure 10–18. Relationship of centric relation to centric occlusion. (See text.)

Working and Balancing from Centric Relation

1. With the condylar elements unlocked, make right and left lateral movements from centric relation, first observing the working side and then the balancing side.
2. Do premature contacts act as interferences in both working and balancing? If so, what supporting cusps related to centric stops are involved?

_____

_____

3. With No. 28 gauge green wax (or blue articulating paper or both) locate the interference on the balancing side. Check the wax as well as the natural teeth. Indicate location of balancing interferences.

Summary Analysis

1. What changes have to be made in the natural dentition (casts)?

_____

2. What changes might then be anticipated in the waxing?

_____

_____

Unit 10 Exercises

1. Unlock the condylar stops and raise the incisal guidance pin. Move the upper member of the articulator so that there is a movement from centric relation to centric occlusion. Repeat, using articulating paper. Observe the direction of slide starting with centric relation and going to centric occlusion.

2. Using the letters CRC indicate on Figure 10–19 where centric relation contact now occurs without an occlusal adjustment.

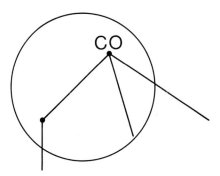

Figure 10–19.

3. The movement from centric relation to centric occlusion is called _____
   _____ .

4. Indicate on Figure 10–19 where CRC should be with the removal of the premature contacts.

5. In the natural dentition, what is meant by the concept of making centric relation and centric occlusion "coincide"?

   _____

6. If an occlusal adjustment were carried out, what would the vertical dimension at centric relation be?

   _____

7. If the incisal pin in contact with the incisal table establishes the vertical dimension when the casts are mounted, after the occlusal interferences in

   centric relation are removed, the incisal pin should be _____

   _____ .

8. If a restoration is waxed in centric occlusion on an articulator that cannot be set for centric relation, what error will result?

   _____

9. If a restoration is waxed on an articulator that does not allow lateral movements, what errors may result?

_____

10. If an occlusal adjustment is not done to eliminate premature contacts in centric relation and balancing interferences, what problems may occur?

_____

Unit 10 Test

1. The modified waxing technique used here is very similar to what has been called the:

   a. wax-added method
   b. add on method
   c. wax-to-wax method
   d. Payne method
   e. all of the above

2. The technique is principally useful for:

   a. one-to-two teeth occlusion
   b. cusp-to-fossa and cusp-to-marginal ridge occlusion
   c. a and b
   d. cusp to fossa occlusion
   e. a, b, and d

3. What parts of the waxed tooth should make contact when the teeth are in centric?

   a. supporting cusp tips
   b. centric stops on teeth opposing the centric stops
   c. a and b
   d. axial surfaces of maxillary molars
   e. a, b, and d

4. In balancing movement, which of the following should make contact?

   a. buccal cusps of mandibular molars
   b. lingual cusps of maxillary molars
   c. a and b
   d. no posterior teeth
   e. a, b, and d

5. The first wax to be added should be:

   a. supporting cusp tips
   b. nonsupporting cusp tips
   c. centric stops in fossa
   d. triangular ridges

6. The lingual concavities of anterior maxillary teeth are determined by:

   a. condylar inclination (mainly)
   b. mandibular movement (only)
   c. posterior guidance (molars)
   d. tooth guidance (mainly)
   e. none of the above

   The following statements describe the functional criteria for the mandibular movements listed in questions 7–9.

   a. no anterior tooth contacts
   b. no posterior tooth contacts
   c. either the canine or several teeth contact on the working side
   d. no posterior tooth contacts on the balancing side
   e. no posterior tooth contacts on the working side

7. Balancing movement:

   a   b   c   d   e

8. Working movement:

   a   b   c   d   e

9. Protrusive movement:

   a   b   c   d   e

10. Posterior centric stops:

    1. are best located to be in the long axis of maxillary posterior teeth
    2. are best located in the central fossa of maxillary posterior teeth
    3. are best located on flat areas of restoration of mandibular posterior teeth
    4. may not be enlarged by grinding
    5. may be enlarged by grinding

       a. 2 and 4
       b. 1 and 2
       c. 1, 2, 3, and 5
       d. 2, 3, 4, and 5
       e. 1, 2, 3, 4, and 5

11. In the wax-added technique of waxing, that part of the wax instrument that is heated first to pick up wax is:

    a. the tip of the blade
    b. the middle of the blade
    c. the shank of the blade
    d. the full blade and shank
    e. b and c

12. After wax has been picked up on the instrument, the blade is returned to the flame and:

    a. the wax is flamed
    b. the middle of the blade is heated
    c. the shank is heated
    d. the tip is heated
    e. a and d

13. When an instrument is heated at the middle of the blade that is parallel to the table top and has wax in the middle of the blade, the wax will flow:

   a. toward the shank
   b. toward the tip of the blade
   c. a and b
   d. toward the flame
   e. a, b, and d

14. Centric stops are sometimes referred to as centric cusps when related to supporting cusps. Terms that are used for the maxillary buccal and the mandibular lingual cusps are:

   a. shear cusps
   b. noncentric cusps
   c. a and b
   d. supporting cusps
   e. a, b, and d

15. The dusting powder used for checking occlusal relations is:

   a. zinc stearate
   b. zinc carbonate
   c. calcium carbonate
   d. diatomaceous earth
   e. none of the above

Unit 11

Occlusal Splint (Bite Plane)

An occlusal splint, or occlusal bite plane splint, is an acrylic intraoral device used for occlusal therapy. As discussed here and elsewhere, an occlusal splint is used for a number of reasons, including the control of night grinding (bruxism). For this reason such splints are often called night guards. The most common name for the devices used to control injury in a contact sport is mouth guards; these are made of a soft pliable material.

Although the pliable mouth guard* is advocated for contact sports, it is not advocated for the control of "night grinding." The term night guard should be replaced by the term occlusal splint or occlusal bite plane splint. Unfortunately, the term night guard is entrenched in the language and may be difficult to eradicate. Unlike "night guard," the term occlusal splint does not describe a device used exclusively for the treatment of nocturnal bruxism. Thus the term occlusal splint is more universal than night guard and describes an appliance that also promotes occlusal stability and may be used for purposes other than control of night grinding. The objective of this unit is to describe the theoretical and practical aspects of an occlusal bite plane splint.

INTRODUCTION: UNIT OBJECTIVES AND READING

Several behavioral objectives are desired for this unit. Some require that the reading be done; this should take place before study of this unit is begun.

A. Objectives
1. Be able to distinguish between an occlusal splint and a "night guard."
2. Be able to name and discuss indications for treatment using an occlusal splint.
3. Be able to discuss the major goal behind the existing concepts of use and design of occlusal splints.
4. Be able to discuss the principal requirements for minimizing disturbances to the masticatory system with the use of an occlusal splint.
5. Be able to discuss the physical requirements of an occlusal splint.

B. Reading
Kobleleski, W. C., III, and deBoever, J.: Influence of occlusal splints on jaw position and musculature in patients with temporomandibular joint dysfunction. J. Prosthet. Dent. 33:321, 1974.

RATIONALE FOR OCCLUSAL SPLINTS

Ideas on the design of an occlusal bite plane splint vary from one school, clinician, and author to the next. Depending upon the rationale for its use, concepts of a well-made splint range from appliances made of soft resilient material to metal, from a smooth hard surface to one with maximum cusp indentation, and from contacts on all the teeth to contacts on only the anterior or posterior teeth. The reasons for using splints vary from splinting teeth to moving teeth, from preventing or curing bruxism to curing headaches, and from preventing tooth abrasion or wear, to myofunctional therapy.

---

*One of the principal drawbacks of the mouth guard is the use of sheets of material that have the same thickness from the incisors to molars. This induces grinding on molars where contact is made first and also causes torque on the joints. Wedge-shaped sheets could solve the material problem.

The common thread that connects the different concepts of rationale and design for an occlusal splint, regardless of its name, is the idea of keeping the teeth apart. How this goal is accomplished, and what purpose it is to serve, are the major sources of differences in the design and use of occlusal splints.

GOALS FOR SPLINT THERAPY

The major goal for the occlusal splint is *to isolate the contact relations of the teeth from the masticatory system without introducing disturbing influences related to the presence of the splint itself.* This goal is purely hypothetical, for it is impossible to isolate the contact relations entirely or to introduce such a foreign object into the mouth without producing disturbing influences. However, as a treatment goal, it is quite practical to control temporomandibular joint–muscle pain dysfunction related to disturbing contact relations of the teeth by the use of a properly designed occlusal splint. Without the goal, regardless of how hypothetical it may appear to be, it is entirely impractical to design an appliance that will successfully minimize unfavorable contact relations and at the same time have minimal disturbing feedback to the masticatory system.

Treatment Effectiveness

The treatment effectiveness of an occlusal splint is related to how well the goal has been met of isolating unfavorable occlusal contact relations without interjecting new disturbing influences to the masticatory system. Assuming that the splint is to be used (1) to treat functional temporomandibular joint–muscle disturbances or (2) to provide for proper registration of centric relation for restorative purposes, the goal of minimizing disturbing occlusal contacts could be met by wiring the teeth (jaws) together. However, this is not a practical method, nor is it highly effective. At least, the use of an acrylic splint between the contacting surfaces of the teeth is practical and is very effective. The minimization of disturbing influences to the masticatory system from the splint itself is the most difficult part of the goal to meet.

Minimizing Disturbing Influences from Splints

The principal requirements for minimizing disturbing influences are (1) to provide for freedom from interference to any movement when the teeth are in contact with the splint, (2) to allow for closure of the mandible into a stable contact relation without interference, (3) to allow for a vertical dimension that can be adapted to readily at a "rest position," (4) to allow for lip seal if possible, (5) not to interfere with swallowing, (6) not to interfere with speaking, (7) not to interfere with the buccal mucosa, and (8) to provide for the most favorable esthetics under the circumstances.

THE OCCLUSAL BITE PLANE SPLINT

The type of splint to be discussed is shown in Figure 11–1. It fits all the occlusal surfaces of the maxillary teeth and is held in place by the acrylic fitting into undercuts in the buccal interproximal dental areas. It is made of heat-cured clear acrylic. The occlusal splint has a smooth surface, makes contact with the mandibular supporting cusps, and has cuspid guidance. The cuspid guidance disoccludes supporting cusp contact almost as soon as lateral or protrusive mandibular movements are made (Fig. 11–1B). The reason for such disclusion is to eliminate as much feedback as possible from contacts away from the "splint centric." Eccentric contacts on a splint can and do cause asynchronous muscle activity and tend to aggravate bruxism. Inasmuch as the treatment of bruxism and temporomandibular joint–muscle pain dysfunction is the primary function of the splint, then eccentric interferences or contacts (especially balancing) or both are avoided in the occlusal splint by use of cuspid-guided disclusion.

PHYSICAL REQUIREMENTS OF AN OCCLUSAL SPLINT

The physical requirements of the occlusal splint are (1) coverage of all the maxillary teeth; (2) smooth, flat occlusal contact surfaces for all mandibular supporting cusps; (3) freedom in "centric"; (4) cuspid

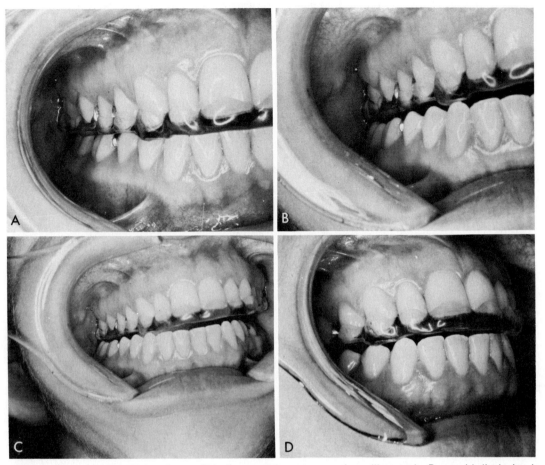

Figure 11-1. Occlusal bite plane splint. *A,* complete coverage of maxillary arch; *B,* cuspid disclusion in lateral; *C,* no balancing contacts; *D,* no incisal contacts in protrusive.

guidance for protrusive and lateral movements; (5) no incisal guidance; (6) occlusal stability; (7) an economical material used for construction that has moderate shock from tooth impact and is easy to adjust; (8) minimal contact vertical dimension; (9) minimum bulk; and (10) esthetic acceptability. Some of these requirements have higher priority than others and for a given occlusal splint, compromises must be made. Items numbered 1, 2, 3, 4, 5, and 6 are higher in priority than other items.

Coverage of Maxillary Teeth

The occlusal splint is placed on the maxillary arch primarily because less bulk is needed to maintain it there, it can be retained better, and it makes a better appearance there. The splint can usually be made with less horizontal overlap, especially in the anterior region, when it is made on the maxillary arch. Often the

maxillary splint can be hidden behind the upper lip, can be made thin enough to allow normal or nearly normal speaking, and can provide for a lip seal. The extension of the splint onto the palatal gingiva provides added strength against warpage, and when interproximal tissues have been lost with periodontal disease, phonetic problems are minimized. A lower splint may be required in an Angle Class III with complete lingual version of the maxillary teeth.

Smooth, Flat Contact Surfaces

A splint with a smooth, flat surface is in distinct contrast to one with cusp indentations, which may be a cause for "playing" (with the rough areas) and in effect may trigger bruxism. All surfaces where supporting cusps make contact must be smooth and flat, except the surface where the cuspid makes contact. Here the surface plane changes from flat to inclined in order to produce disclusion of all cusp contacts other than the cuspid. Smoothness of non-contact areas is also important because patients tend to play with rough areas with their tongue.

Freedom in "Centric"

The freedom in "centric" that is desired is an area corresponding to both centric relation and centric occlusion, but perhaps more appropriately a comfort zone for the "splint centric" at the time of relating the mandible to the maxilla in mounting the casts. In effect, it may not be possible to obtain centric relation during functional disturbances. Because the exact location — vertical or horizontal — of "centric" (splint centric) is not known, a small (.05 × 0.5 mm) flat area is provided for freedom of contact before cuspid guidance takes over. Furthermore, contacts on closure in swallowing vary with head position and other factors. Thus precise closure to a point does not occur. Interference to closure about "splint centric" is to be avoided.

As the temporomandibular joint–muscle pain dysfunction abates, the mandible may adjust its position and the splint surface may have to be adjusted by grinding to accommodate the new mandibular position. Adjustment of the splint must be made to accommodate mandibular movement. New contact areas on the splint must be flat, and freedom must be provided for cusp movements, including movement by the cuspid where the cuspid rise requires special attention to freedom in splint centric.

Cuspid Guidance

In order to prevent protrusive and balancing interferences, a cuspid rise is placed in the splint. In the normal arrangement of teeth, cuspid disclusion in lateral movement takes place between the distal cusp ridge of the mandibular cuspid and the mesial cusp ridge of the maxillary cuspid. However, in protrusive excursions of the mandible, the disclusion occurs because of contact between the mesial cusp ridge (and buccal axial surface) of the mandibular first premolar and the distal cusp

ridge (and distal slope) of the triangular ridge of the maxillary cuspid. This contact relationship and disclusion of posterior teeth by the cuspid does not mean that simultaneous contact of the incisors may not occur at the same time in protrusive. It probably does occur solely on the incisors in many instances in protrusive. However, the function of the splint is to avoid all protrusive and lateral contacts that could act or have acted as occlusal interferences or as a trigger for bruxism. On the splint, protrusive as well as lateral disclusion occurs on the mandibular cuspid.

No Incisal Guidance

Probably the most important deterrent to the use of incisal guidance is the response of the muscles to its presence and the related tendency of patients to continue to grind their teeth when an incisal guidance is present. Occlusal splints are much more effective without incisal guidance. Only when other influences that are jeopardizing the effectiveness of the splint outweigh the drawbacks of using incisal guidance should incisal guidance be considered. As will be discussed later, an increased vertical dimension due to the splint is seldom a clinical problem, but some incisal contact may be necessary to avoid a gross exaggeration of the cuspid guidance that would be required to completely eliminate the edge-to-edge type of contact of the incisors.

Incisal guidance should be used only when cuspid guidance would result in a gross or disturbing increase in the vertical dimension. This could be the case not only with a deep impinging overbite but also with an exaggerated curve of Spee. Under such circumstances the incisal guidance may be used in the late stages of cuspid guidance to continue posterior disclusion. However, the general rule is: *Do not use incisal guidance.*

It is easier to develop guidance solely on the mandibular cuspid than for a whole range of incisal guidance areas. From a clinical standpoint it is difficult with a deep overbite to avoid "entrapment" of the mandibular incisors behind an incisal guidance. Also, as dysfunction subsides and as mandibular repositioning occurs, adjustment of the incisal guidance is far more difficult than adjustment of a cuspid guidance.

Occlusal Stability

The term occlusal stability is used here to mean several things. First, it refers to freedom from any tendency the mandible may have to move from a less well supported position to a better supported position on the splint. For example, when the mandible makes closure, most of the mandibular supporting cusp tips should make simultaneous contact with the splint; aside from cuspid contact guidance on mandibular closure, there should not be premature contacts by one or more supporting cusp tips to produce a slide into a more stable position of multiple contacts.

Second, the term occlusal stability refers to an absence of drifting, shifting, extruding or other movement of the teeth related to the design of the splint. For example, failure to provide for adequate centric stops will lead to extrusion of the teeth and development of interferences. Some splints (viz., Sved) have no posterior contacts and should be used only for short periods of time because posterior teeth tend to extrude.

Third, the term refers to an absence of "rocking" when the supporting cusps make contact with the splint on mandibular closure. When fully seated, the splint should not "rock" when pressure is applied at any point on its surface. The absence of rock is a function of adequate seating of the device; it is not dependent except indirectly on retention from undercuts. Retention from undercuts is primarily for the purpose of guarding against dislodgement by suction and gravity.

Fourth, occlusal stability means that the device will not cause orthodontic movement of the teeth. For example, there should be no lingual or labial pressure on the maxillary central incisors when the splint is being worn. Also, centric stops should not be placed on inclined planes or axial surfaces of supporting cusp tips.

Fifth, the term is used to mean a relationship between the components of the masticatory system that is conducive to homeostasis of the system.

Splint Material

The perfect material for an occlusal splint has not been found, but heat-cured clear acrylic is the best material available at this time. Patients with bruxism will "chew up" a soft material and in the process will not get the hoped-for relief from dysfunctional disturbances. Metal appliances, especially those made of chrome cobalt, are extremely difficult to adjust as mandibular repositioning occurs. In addition, the shock related to occlusal contacts is not deadened with metal as it is with acrylic. Soreness of individual teeth is much more likely to occur with high spots on metal devices than on acrylic. The metal occlusal splint is not feasible to adjust initially in the presence of temporomandibular joint dysfunction and is much more expensive to make than is the acrylic. The advantages of the metal splint are mostly dimensional — it can be made thinner than the occlusal splint made of acrylic and will not distort as easily as a plastic splint.

Contact Vertical Dimension

There is no available scientific evidence for producing an occlusal splint with a specific contact vertical dimension. However, clinical experience suggests that this dimension should be kept at a minimum, but consistent with other requirements. A splint that has a large anterior dimension interferes with lip seal, makes speaking difficult, often causes excessive salivation, and is esthetically unacceptable to most patients. Such a splint may also interfere with sleep.

A reasonable encroachment on the freeway space may be adapted to quite readily on a temporary basis by some patients; others cannot adjust. The failure to adjust may be seen as failure to wear the splint, failure to obtain relief of temporomandibular joint–muscle pain dysfunction, and an aggravation of symptoms and abnormal muscle patterns, especially in swallowing. If a patient with a splint has difficulty in swallowing, this is because the vertical dimension of the splint is too great or the splint is too bulky, or both, and there is unacceptable encroachment on the tongue space.

A patient who is a "tongue thruster," or has an anterior open bite or both problems, may fail to adapt readily to an encroachment on the tongue space. The superimposed muscle activity related to such adaptation may aggravate an already existing hypertonicity of the masticatory muscles.

Several factors determine contact vertical dimension. The anterior thickness of the splint is determined mostly by the minimum thickness of the splint at the most distal supporting cusp contact. It may also be determined by other factors such as the amount of freedom in centric desired, curve of Spee, malposed teeth, condylar guidance, and the amount of grinding that might be expected on the splint. These factors will be considered in more detail under the heading *Biomechanics of an Occlusal Splint.*

The vertical dimension should not be at the point of a click or trip in a joint. It should not be so great as to interfere with swallowing or sleeping.

The acrylic should not be less than 1 mm in thickness over all areas of functional contact with supporting cusps. It may be less than a millimeter over nonsupporting cusps and over the gingival tissue.

USE AND MAINTENANCE OF THE OCCLUSAL SPLINT

The manifold uses of the occlusal splint will not be discussed at this time, but a few concepts about their use will be presented as an introduction to the reasons for fabricating an occlusal splint. The occlusal splint is used for the treatment of temporomandibular joint–muscle pain dysfunction, as a diagnostic device to rule out or verify occlusion as a cause of obscure pain or symptoms of unknown origin, and as an aid in registering centric relation for restorative purposes. The exact details of these uses have been discussed elsewhere.

Of interest at this time is the question of when to use a splint — before or after an occlusal adjustment or even in relation to an adjustment. Usually the splint is made and used before the occlusal adjustment in cases in which the adjustment cannot be done adequately because of an inability to obtain centric relation or when the patient has a long history of prior treatments and adjustments that have been inadequate. As soon as practical after completion of splint therapy or during therapy if necessary, the occlusal adjustment is done. After the adjustment the patient may or may not have to use the splint periodically.

Inasmuch as bruxism may be initiated by psychic as well as local occlusal factors, the recurrence of bruxism and related temporomandibular joint symptoms may accompany new bouts of psychic stress. Under such conditions, and even though an adjustment has been done, a patient may need to use the splint periodically, provided that the splint still fits after not having been used for a time. Acrylic splints should be stored in water or at 100 per cent humidity.

In order to register the relationship of the mandible to the maxilla to carry out restorative treatment, it may be necessary to have the patient wear a splint for a period of time. This is so that the occlusal adjustment can be done correctly; otherwise the adjustment would be impossible because of muscle hypertonicity. After the splint is used, the occlusion can be adjusted more effectively and then the relationship of the mandible to the hinge axis may be registered adequately so that the restorative procedures can be done correctly on an articulator.

BIOMECHANICS OF AN OCCLUSAL SPLINT

An occlusal splint is a mechanical device that has several influences on the masticatory system. The biological effects are mediated by the mechanics of the action of the splint. The effects may be related to physiological, anatomical, psychological, and physical factors that are direct and indirect responses to the presence of the splint. The elements of these responses are largely interpretations by the clinician of the effects that the splint has on a patient's symptoms and the patient's perception of the nature of the changes that may or may not have occurred. In any case, the splint is expected to be comfortable, unobtrusive, and acceptable to the patient as treatment modality. It is also expected that unhindered mandibular movement and tooth contact with the splint will occur or the splint will not be effective, and may even cause or aggravate dysfunction. The biomechanical factors in the design of a splint to be considered at this time include vertical dimension, cuspid guidance, and peripheral contours.

Vertical Dimension

The determination of vertical dimension of the splint should not be done without considering the patient. Although they will not be discussed here, certain characteristics of the patient can be used to modify conclusions about vertical dimension. Lip seal, freeway space, swallowing and sleeping habits, speaking, and psychological aspects may all be important. However, at this time the general principle outlined previously will be used: *Keep the vertical dimension as minimal as might be consistent with a smooth, flat surface and with other requirements of an interference-free device.*

The basic idea of the splint is to isolate the disturbing presence of the occlusion. Do not substitute one set of disturbing influences for another — that is, do not design a splint with occlusal interferences such as one with rough areas for the patient to "play with" with the teeth. The determination of vertical dimension is controlled from a mechanical standpoint at the most distal mandibular molar. The anterior opening would be greater with a flat, straight buccal lingual splint plane (Fig. 11–2A,B) than with a recessed plane (Fig. 11–2C). Although the design in Figure 11–2A is preferred, use of that shown in Figure 11–2B may be required because of lingual tipping, and it may be necessary to use that design shown in Figure 11–2C because of a very small vertical dimension required for speaking problems.

The extent to which the contact plane

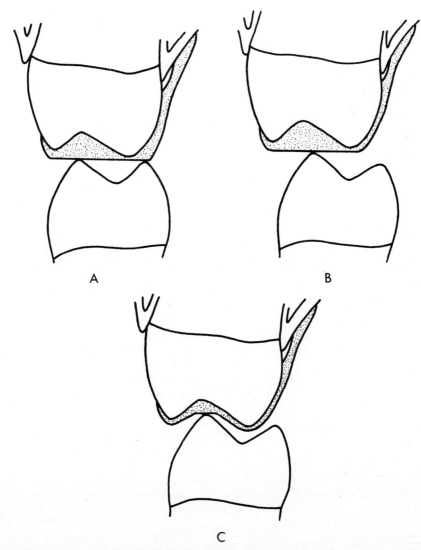

Figure 11–2. Occlusal bite plane splint. *A,* contacts on both buccal and lingual cusps if a balancing interference does not result; *B,* contacts only on buccal cusps with lingual tipping of posterior teeth; *C,* recessed contacts where vertical dimension is critical for speaking.

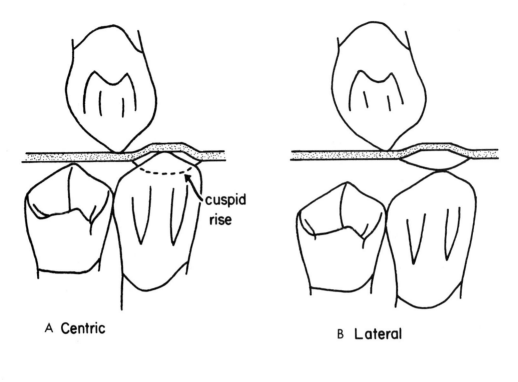

A Centric   B Lateral

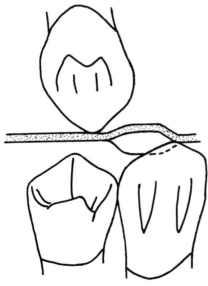

C Protrusive

Figure 11–3. Cuspid rise on splint. *A,* position of cuspid rise in centric; *B,* position for lateral movements; *C,* position in protrusive. Recessed area for cuspid in centric occlusion depends on vertical dimension desired for splint.

Illustration continued on opposite page

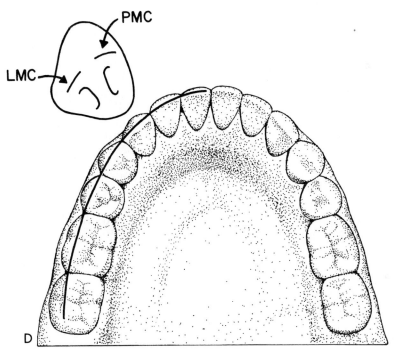

Figure 11-3. *Continued. D,* lateral cuspid guidance should be on the distal cusp ridge (LMC) and protrusive guidance on the mesial cusp bridge of the mandibular cuspid (PMC).

can be recessed depends on physical as well as physiological factors. There must be sufficient clearance (distance) for the cusps to avoid contact in "centric" as well as in various excursions. There must be room for freedom in centric, not only on the posterior teeth but also at the cuspid guidance area and at the incisor area.

Vertical dimension is often a compromise between cuspid rise height and the need to avoid balancing interferences (and contacts) and protrusive contacts caused by third molars and an exaggerated curve of Spee.

Cuspid Guidance

Cuspid guidance must be considered in lateral, lateral protrusive, and protrusive movements from "splint centric" outward to near the border of the splint. The border

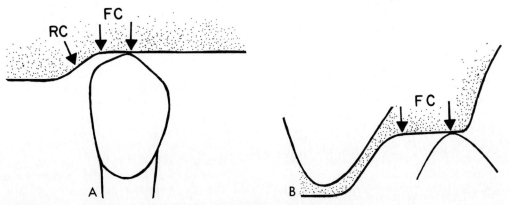

Figure 11-4. Freedom in splint centric. *A,* freedom in splint centric (FC) between arrows; *RC,* cuspid rise. *B,* transition from FC to cuspid rise is smooth and continuous.

movement for the splint should not be farther than that which exists for end-to-end occlusion without the splint. The mandibular cuspid provides the disclusion in protrusive, not the bicuspid (Fig. 11–3). For a cuspid bruxing habit, this change in position is often critical in muscle function. The height of the cuspid guidance in the end-to-end position (border position) should just be sufficient to provide posterior disclusion and, within reason, anterior disclusion. The height should be slightly greater in the waxed splint to allow for adjustment and polishing of the acrylic.

Use. The principal use of cuspid guidance is to control balancing side contacts in lateral movements and posterior contacts in protrusive movements. An aggravated curve of Spee, balancing interferences, and a deep vertical overlap all require an increased vertical dimension of the splint. The absence of cuspid guidance contributes to continual bruxism. Significant to the success of splint therapy is the correct lateral placement of the cuspid rise. Its placement must take into account any lateral slide that is present in centric.

Freedom in Centric. Freedom in centric must be provided at the point of contact of the mandibular cuspid on the splint. Freedom in centric should be 0.5×0.5 mm. Such an area (Fig. 11–4) is difficult to produce in wax without using an articulator with an incisal pin and table designed to provide the freedom required. Even though such an articulator is used when the splint is placed in the mouth, adjustment to freedom in centric is necessary.

Pattern of Movements. When the surface of a waxed splint is dusted with zinc stearate and the cuspid moved into protrusive and straight lateral movements with an incisal guide being used, there should be a pattern shown that demonstrates the paths made by the cuspid. The preferred path pattern should be a V (see Figure 11–5), but this goal is not always attainable because of the position of the lateral incisor. In effect, in protrusive the mesial cusp ridge or cusp tip or both should be making primary contact with the splint (hence the V pattern) rather than with the axial surface of the cusp ridge and cusp tip. The principle of stability involved here is that points (cusp tips) and lines (cusp ridges) are less deflecting and unstable than two

inclined planes (axial surfaces of cuspid against the inclined plane of the cuspid guidance of the splint).

Form of Cuspid Guidance. The form or height of the cuspid guidance will to some extent be determined by the occlusal plane and the vertical dimension. For a deep overbite (vertical overlap) the cuspid rise may start below the surface of the posterior part of the splint, i.e., contacts for posterior teeth. Less vertical overlap could result in a greater vertical dimension of the cuspid rise above the posterior part of the splint. A general principle is: *Use cuspid height principally to disclude posterior contacts in protrusive and lateral movements, and use splint vertical dimension to control the curve of Spee and vertical overlap.* The greater the vertical overlap and curve of Spee (less radius), the greater the vertical dimension for the splint and cuspid rise.

Position of Cuspid Guidance. The position (anteroposterior and lateral) of cuspid guidance is one of the most important aspects of splint design. The general principle to be followed is: *Place the cuspid rise so that in swallowing and on opening and closing, the mandible does not have to adjust laterally to avoid a cuspid rise. Rule: Do not prevent the mandible from moving to a position of least condylar movement.*

Although cuspid guidance is used to cause disclusion in all movements from centric to avoid balancing contacts, posterior contacts, and incisal guidance, such guidance should be unobtrusive. It should not guide to pain or dysfunction, but to the point of minimum movement on the side of pain. It should allow the mandible to close into a stable position most efficiently and effortlessly at any time. It should not force the mandible into a retruded or retruded-lateral position. For example, a painful temporomandibular joint–muscle dysfunction on the left side often results in a limitation of movement of that joint. The position of the cuspid guidance should not prevent such limitation — it should not cause condylar shifting to avoid the cuspid rise and in effect prevent the condyle from functioning in a position of minimum movement on the left side.

The position of the cuspid guidance, as well as the vertical dimension of the

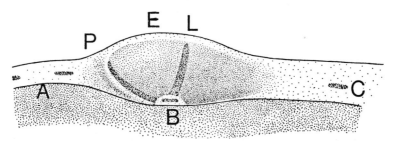

Figure 11–5. Cuspid rise–movement paths. Incisor contact area *(A)*; freedom in centric *(B)*; posterior contacts *(C)*; lateral *(L)* protrusive *(P)* area of contact is continuous *(E)*.

splint, may require changing during splint therapy. Changes in temporomandibular joint muscle function can produce differential alterations in vertical dimension (side-to-side, anterior, posterior) as well as lateral and rotational movements. Small changes in yaw, pitch, and roll of the mandible may be very significant.

Protrusive Guidance

There are two other major elements to be considered in the protrusive guidance: the curve of Spee and freedom of incisal guidance. Assuming the incisal inclination to be constant, the less the horizontal overlap, the more acute the angle of the cuspid rise must be to prevent incisal contact with the splint. At a point of putting most, if not all, of the guidance on axial surfaces of the mandibular cuspid, and at the point of having an inclination of the incisal guide table greater than 60°, a greater opening of the vertical should be considered to avoid problems connected with cuspid entrapment. Figure 11–6 shows failure to provide freedom in centric and an entrapment of the cuspid on an inclined plane.

As the mandible is moved into a protrusive position, the cuspid guidance should take over the guidance beyond the area of freedom in centric (Fig. 11–7*B,C*), and there should be no contact with the anterior part of the splint (Fig. 11–7*D*). When there is hardly any vertical overlap, beyond freedom in centric contact (FC), the splint should fall away rapidly to avoid any incisal contact or guidance (Fig. 11–8).

In those patients in whom there are no natural teeth that may be used for cuspid guidance (missing teeth, loose teeth, sore teeth), it may be appropriate to use incisal guidance rather than open the vertical to

an end-to-end relation. Each case must be evaluated clinically for the appropriate method.

Borders of the Splint

Using the principle of cuspid guidance in lateral and protrusive positions, the splint material should not extend more than about 1 mm beyond the surface of the maxillary teeth that are being covered. For example, the facial edge of the splint should follow the contours of the cusp tip (Fig. 11–9). It should not extend outward, have a sharp edge, or present a bulky profile to the buccal and labial mucosa.

The contour on the palatal side should follow closely the anatomical contours of the gingiva. There should be no impingement on the free gingival margin.

The palatal edge should blend in with the rugae and taper into the distal maxillary molar soon after the second premolar or first molar. The edge of the splint should not cross rugae. The thickness of the splint adjacent to the second molars and behind the incisors should be minimal. If necessary, stainless steel wire may be used to provide added strength to the acrylic.

Occlusal Plane

For expediency the various problems encountered in the design of an occlusal splint have been related to four types of occlusal relations. The classification (Fig. 11–10) is not considered to be exhaustive, analytical or critical, but merely a frame of reference about which to discuss the design of splints. Any one of the types may be made more complex by individual variations in the position of the teeth. The

INCORRECT CUSPID RISE

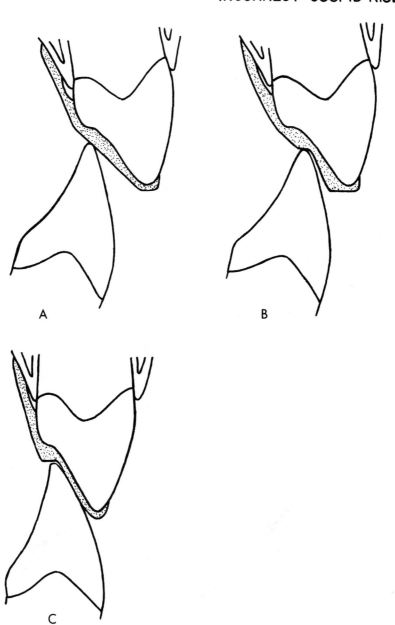

Figure 11–6. Incorrect cuspid rise. *A,* centric stop on incline plane, no freedom in splint centric, unstable position; *B, C,* cuspid entrapment with guidance on axial surface.

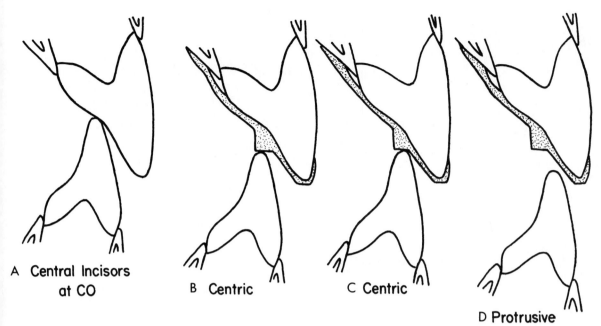

Figure 11–7. Protrusive guidance. *A*, centric occlusion; *B*, splint centric relation contact; *C*, splint centric on tapping; *D*, cuspid disclusion, no incisal guidance.

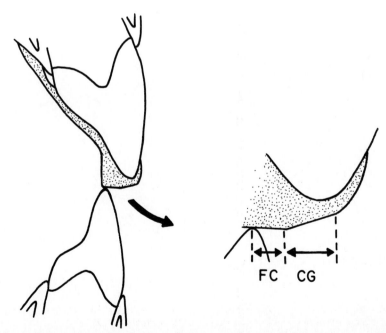

Figure 11–8. Absence of incisal guidance. *FC*, freedom in splint centric; *CG*, zone of cuspid guidance; arrow indicates disclusion by cuspid.

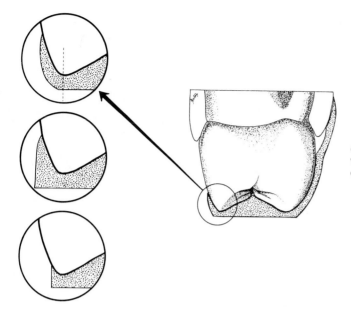

Figure 11–9. Border of splint. Border of splint should be rounded and extend well beyond the tip of the cusp. Correct contour is indicated by arrow.

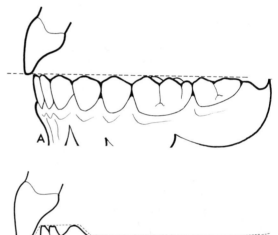

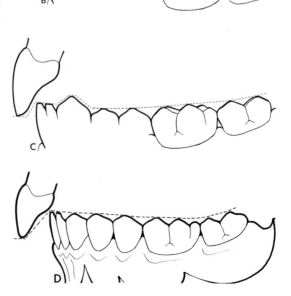

Figure 11–10. Occlusal plane. Types of occlusal plane and effect on splint design. *A,* type I, *B,* type II, *C,* type III, *D,* type IV.

broken line is the contact area for the supporting cusps of the mandibular teeth. The position of the maxillary central incisor may be moved anteriorly or posteriorly to describe the degree of horizontal overlap.

The occlusal plane of Type I splint is virtually straight with no significant overlap of the incisors (Fig. 11–10A). The vertical dimension is determined principally by the cusp height–fossa depth of the distal molar. If an attempt is made to make the buccolingual plane flat, there may be excessive height of the cuspid guidance and of the splint at the first mandibular premolar supporting cusps. Even when the curve of Wilson is not excessive and the condylar guidance reasonable (20° to 30°), the thickness of the splint and height of the cuspid may be excessive in Type I cases. In effect, the use of the flat buccal-lingual plane is sometimes not possible in Type I cases and the centric stop must be placed below the height of the buccal and lingual cusps, as shown in Figure 11–2C.

The occlusal plane of Type II (Fig. 11–10B) is characterized by a moderate vertical overlap of the incisors; the mandibular cuspids and incisors are above the occlusal plane of the molars and premolars, and there is only a slight curve of Spee. The vertical overlap tends to mask the thickness of the splint. It is not possible to have the cusp tips of the mandibular teeth occlude on the same plane. The fact that the heights of the incisors and the cuspid are essentially the same allows the lateral cuspid guidance to be less than in Type I cases, but requires a greater protrusive cuspid guidance to prevent incisal contact in protrusive and lateral protrusive. Unless the curve of Spee is exaggerated at the second molar, the buccal lingual plane is usually flat in Type II cases. The most difficult problem with a Type II case is usually the prevention of incisal contact in protrusive without having an excessive cuspid guidance.

The occlusal plane of Type III (Fig. 11–10C) is characterized by the high position of the mandibular cuspid. Although the depth of the cuspid stop into the splint is great, the relationship of the incisors allows for a cuspid guidance with minimum height above the level of the posterior occlusal plane. Even with a sharp curve of Spee at the molar, the thickness of the splint may be minimized.

The main characteristic of the Type IV occlusal plane (Fig. 11–10D) is the extensive vertical overlap and low position of the mandibular cuspid. The posterior vertical should not be raised to prevent incisal contact or guidance — that is, raised beyond the minimal buccal lingual flat plane. In a Type IV occlusal plane it is difficult to prevent the cuspid guidance from being quite high in avoiding incisal contact or guidance. In the event there is also an exaggerated curve of Spee at the distal mandibular molar, the vertical dimension may have to be increased at the molar. This increase would necessitate a thicker splint.

Vertical Dimension and Cuspid Guidance

Contact vertical dimension and the height of cuspid guidance present both physiologic and esthetic problems. In most instances both the vertical dimension and the height of the cuspid guidance should be minimal. However, in some instances, especially in deep overbite and a suspected loss of vertical dimension, the vertical dimension of the splint may work best at 6 to 7 mm. A patient who bruxes on a cuspid may find the cuspid rise in the same attractive position to continue bruxing. Both vertical and lateral positioning should be set to avoid such a position.

MOUNTING CASTS

The mandibular cast that is to be used in the fabrication of a splint may be mounted in three ways: (1) centric relation, (2) centric occlusion, and (3) in an open vertical approximating the vertical dimension to be used for the splint. The method to be used depends on several factors.

Note: It is possible to fabricate a splint on a single unmounted maxillary cast. However, the use of quick-cure acrylic and extensive intraoral adjustment is not recommended except for emergencies.

Methods of Mounting the Mandibular Cast

Centric Relation. The mandibular cast should be mounted in centric relation in all cases if possible inasmuch as vertical dimension is increased significantly for the splint on the articulator. However, in the presence of temporomandibular joint–muscle pain dysfunction, obtaining a correct centric relation registration is often practically impossible.

The maxillary cast should be keyed and painted with a separating medium if a split cast technique is to be used. The split cast method has limited value for mounting in centric occlusion or open vertical.

Centric Occlusion. The mandibular cast may be mounted in centric occlusion if (1) there is a small discrepancy between centric relation and centric occlusion, (2) there is no significant lateral deviation of the mandible on opening and closing, and (3) there is no significant lateral slide in centric.

Open Vertical. The mandibular cast is mounted at an open vertical if there is a major discrepancy between centric relation and centric occlusion, a significant lateral slide in centric (>0.5 mm), and a significant lateral deviation of the mandible on opening and closing (2.0 mm at 3 to 4 mm vertical). The method is very useful for setting the vertical dimension of the splint to avoid having the thickness of the splint at a point of clicking and tripping of the joint. It is also useful in setting the vertical dimension outside or inside the point of pain brought on by open and closing movements and clenching. The open vertical registration is very useful with both centric relation and centric occlusion registration in setting the position of the cuspid rise when there is a significant lateral deviation of the mandible and lateral slide in centric. This aspect has been discussed under the placement of the cuspid guidance.

PREPARATION FOR WAXING SPLINT

The objective of this section is to provide an initial experience in the design and waxing of an occlusal bite plane splint. The principles for the design of a splint have already been outlined. The initial step in waxing the splint is the setting of the articulator for the correct vertical dimension in centric as well as in lateral excursions.

Setting the Articulator

Set the incisal table, incisal pin, offset pin, and the FC pin to provide a minimum of 0.02″ freedom in centric. Move the upper member into protrusive for slight contact of the anterior teeth. Customize the incisal table if necessary to obtain sufficient guidance when the table is already set at a maximum.

The condylar guidance (C.G.) is set to be reasonably parallel with the occlusal plane (C.G. > 0).

Set the lateral wings for slight clearance of the cuspids in lateral movements from both centric relation and centric occlusion. Make certain that the cuspids make only light contact in lateral excursions. In protrusive, the maxillary cuspid may make light contact with the mandibular first premolar.

At this time, the vertical dimension is increased to the thickness desired for the splint. A simple method is to increase the setting of the offset pin to the point at which an index card can be placed between opposing molars (Fig. 11–11). The separation between the cuspids also has to be considered. In lateral the separation should be equal to one thickness of base plate wax between the cuspids. If necessary, increase the angulation of the lateral wings to prevent the balancing side from making contact when one thickness of base plate wax is present on the occlusal surfaces.

Outline of Coverage

Mark the outline of the splint on the maxillary cast (Fig. 11–12). The extent of

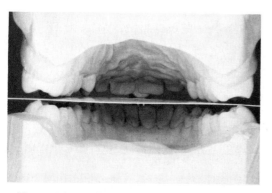

Figure 11–11. Setting articulator. In most instances the degree of opening (vertical) can be set with a card between the posterior teeth.

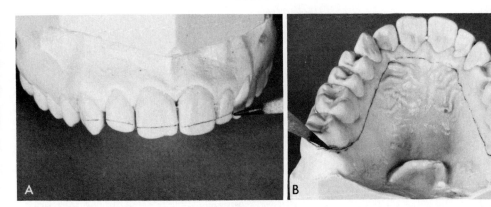

Figure 11–12. Outlining splint coverage. *A,* splint should extend 2–3 mm cervically from the incisal edges; *B,* palatal margins extend to attached gingiva. Margins on distal molars should extend above height of contour on the buccal surfaces.

the splint on the palatal side is determined by the thickness of the gingival margin and the bony contours. The splint should just bridge the free gingival margin and the unattached gingiva, and it should reach the edge of the attached gingiva. Keep the outline just above the height of contour on the facial surfaces of the molar teeth and toward the incisal edges on the incisor teeth.

Block Out Undercuts

Using a thin mix of stone, paint the lingual interproximal areas to block out undercuts (Fig. 11–13). Where deep developmental grooves occur, these should be filled with stone also. If such grooves are not filled, when the wax is replaced with acrylic the splint will not be seated correctly on the teeth in the mouth. Most interproximal undercuts on the facial side should be left for retention. All embrasure areas should be filled. Retention is obtained on the facial surfaces, principally from cuspid to molar teeth, not from incisor interproximal areas. The incisive papilla should be blocked out for relief.

WAXING THE SPLINT

Lock the condylar elements into position. Observe the opening between the anterior teeth and between the posterior teeth. Usually more base plate wax is required in the anterior region than in the posterior area. Using hot water in a bowl or a Bunsen burner, heat two folded layers of

hard pink base plate wax cut to about 1½ inches wide, and mold into a U shape on the maxillary arch cast (Fig. 11–14A). Continue to heat the wax with a torch, lamp, or burner as the wax is adapted to the occlusal and facial surfaces. Trim excess wax outside the pencil mark outline made previously on the maxillary cast. Do most of the trimming while the wax is still heated. Tack peripheral wax to outline the form of the cast with a No. 7 spatula.

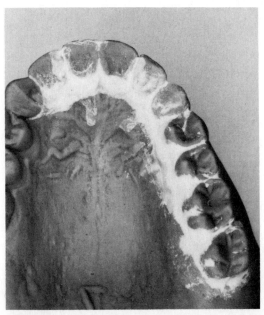

Figure 11–13. Blocking out undercuts. All undercuts on palatal side and embrasures should be blocked out with stone. Also deep developmental grooves must be eliminated. Do not block out interproximal areas on buccal surfaces.

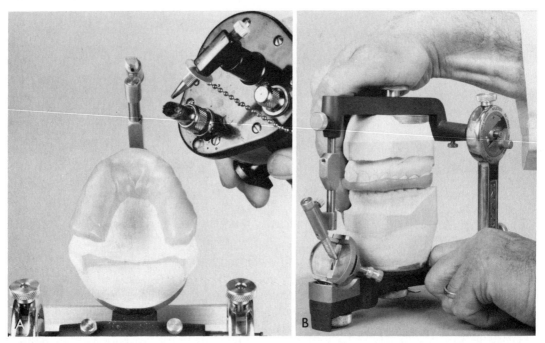

Figure 11–14. Waxing the splint. *A*, two heated layers of base plate wax are adapted to occlusal surfaces; *B*, articulator is closed until contact of incisal pin.

Occlusal Surface

Heat the occlusal surfaces as in Figure 11–14*A* and close the articulator until the incisal pin is in contact with the table (Fig. 11–14*B*). Make sure that mandibular anterior teeth contact on the wax. If no contact is made (Fig. 11–15), trim some of the wax in the posterior area and reheat. Close until all contacts are present. Repeat as

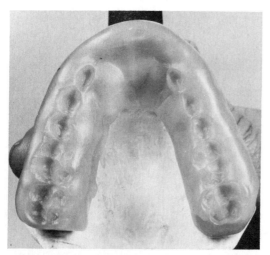

Figure 11–15. Waxing the splint. Indentations should also be present in the area of the incisors; therefore more wax must be added in this area.

often as necessary. When all contacts are present in the wax, trim excess wax and mark contacts with articulating paper (Fig. 11–16). Heat the occlusal surfaces evenly and cut away the excess wax using the marks made by the articulating paper as a guide.

It is not necessary for mandibular lingual cusps to contact the wax in splint centric (Fig. 11–17). However, additional wax may be needed to have centric stops in the anterior region.

Compare the curvature of the wax between the right and left sides at the second molar. The cuspid rise may have to be greater on one side than the other to avoid protrusive or balancing interferences or both. The final shape of the splint lingual to the supporting cusp will depend upon the cuspid rise to be developed for lateral movements. The mandibular buccal cusps should all make contact when there is no unusual cusp height present, and when there is no intrusion or extrusion and/or mesial distal tipping of the teeth.

Facial Surface

Trim the excess wax from the facial surfaces. The wax should be trimmed to

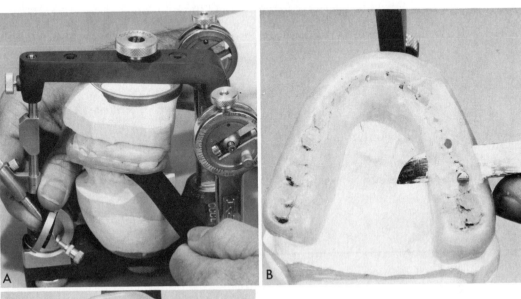

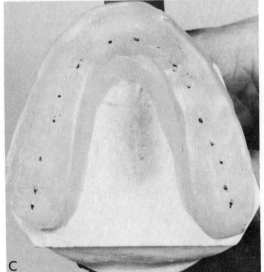

Figure 11–16. Waxing the splint. *A*, use of articulating paper to mark centric stops; *B*, trim wax to level of articulating paper marks; *C*, anterior and posterior marks should be present.

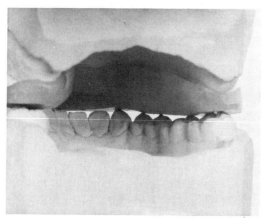

Figure 11–17. Waxing splint. Occlusal contacts are not necessary on the lingual cusps.

the outline made in pencil or slightly beyond to allow for trimming and polishing of the acrylic after processing.

Seal the opening (Fig. 11–18A) between the wax and the cast with a waxing instrument (Fig. 11–18B). The interproximal area shown by the arrow in Figure 11–18A is partially filled with stone except when retention is to be obtained. In some instances the whole interproximal must be filled with wax in order to obtain retention, especially when the gingiva fills the interproximal area, as with children and young adults. Retention may be lost easily if trimming and polishing of the splint are not carefully done.

Cuspid Guidance

With the casts in centric occlusion mark the wax (Fig. 11–19A) to indicate the position in which the cuspid guidance will be placed. Make the line to include lateral as well as protrusive movements. Remember that protrusive guidance should be made on the mesial cusp ridge of the mandibular cuspid (not the first bicuspid) and not on the axial surface of the mandibular cuspid. The proper placement of the anterior guidance in relation to the position of the lateral incisor is essential.

To begin cuspid guidance place a small amount of medium-hard inlay wax or Slaycris wax (Fig. 11–19B) at the periphery of the line that has been drawn on the wax. The wax must be developed so that lateral and all protrusive movements will be guided by the "cuspid rise" so that there are no posterior contacts in protrusive and balancing. If the mounting of the mandibular cast was done by the open vertical method because of a lateral slide in centric, one cuspid rise is placed more laterally than if the cast were mounted in centric occlusion.

Dust the wax surfaces with zinc stearate (Fig. 11–20A). If inlay wax is used, soften the surface of the cuspid guidance with heat first before making excursion movements on the articulator.

Move the upper member of the articulator into straight protrusive and straight lateral positions and observe for posterior contacts (Fig. 11–20B). Observe the marks on the cuspid rise (Fig. 11–20C) in relation to the "occlusal interference" involving posterior teeth. If necessary adjust the lateral wings of the incisal table and add sufficient wax to the cuspid rise to avoid interferences that may be present.

Often overlooked are the marks made on the wax due to an inadequate cuspid rise, especially those made very close to the

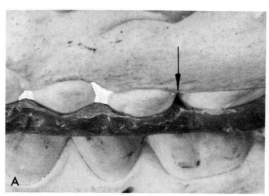
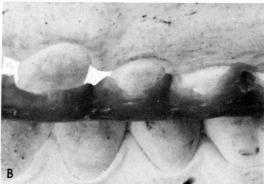

Figure 11–18. Waxing splint. *A,* Interproximal areas (arrow) on buccal are used for retention and should be filled with wax as in *B.* Some areas may be blocked out to control excess retentive areas.

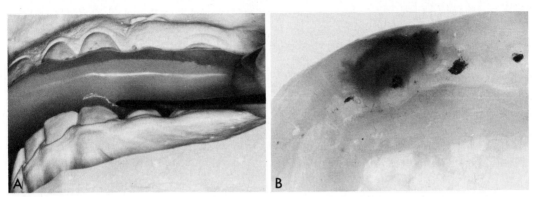

Figure 11-19. Waxing cuspid guidance. *A,* mark area of guidance adjacent to cuspid. Outline should provide for lateral and protrusive disclusion; *B,* add inlay wax to begin cuspid guidance.

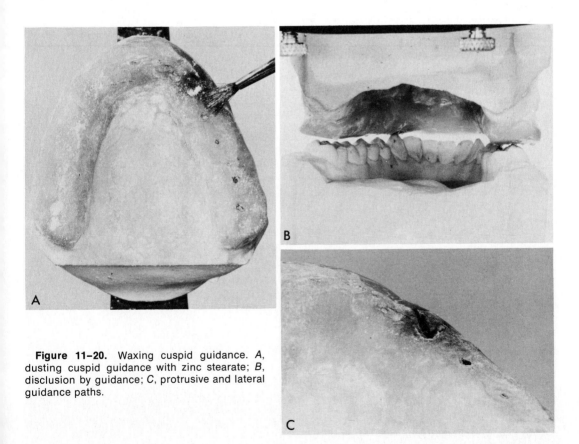

Figure 11-20. Waxing cuspid guidance. *A,* dusting cuspid guidance with zinc stearate; *B,* disclusion by guidance; *C,* protrusive and lateral guidance paths.

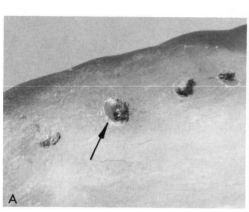
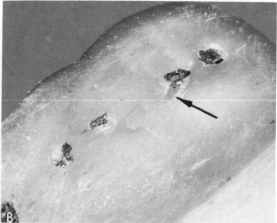

Figure 11–21. Waxing splint. *A,* unwanted "drag" marks in protrusive; *B,* unwanted "drag" marks in balancing. Whole surface needs to be flattened and smoothed.

centric stops (Fig. 11–21*A,B*). There should be no ploughing of the wax in protrusive movements even close to centric stops (Fig. 11–21*A*) nor in the balancing path (Fig. 11–21*B*).

There should be about 0.5 mm freedom in centric developed around the centric stops and around the cuspid contacts in centric. In Figure 11–22 the cuspid guidance has been dusted, then centric stops marked with articulating paper. Note the flat area between the centric stop and the elevation of the cuspid guidance. The movement pattern for all movements from centric occlusion is shown in Figure 11–22*B*. The flat area is for freedom in centric.

Completion of Waxing

After waxing has been completed, dust all surfaces and make all protrusive, lateral movements. There should be no anterior or posterior contacts in lateral or protrusive movements. The cuspid guidance should be just sufficient to avoid posterior and incisor contacts and to allow for some removal (very minimal) of acrylic when the splint is finally smoothed and the acrylic splint is polished (Fig. 11–23).

Summary of Requirements. There should be freedom in centric and continuous contact with the cuspid guidance in lateral and lateral protrusive movements

Figure 11–22. Waxing cuspid guidance. *A,* development of "V" pattern in lateral and protrusive movements; *B,* filling in of "fan" for all protrusive, lateral, and lateral protrusive movements.

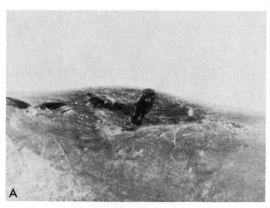
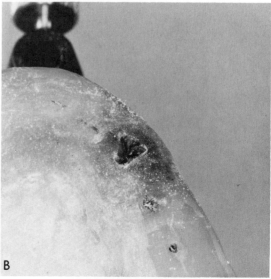

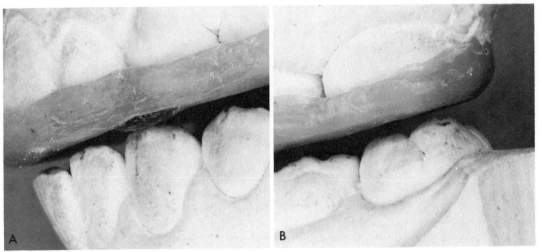

Figure 11–23. Waxing splint. *A,* cuspid disclusion in working; *B,* posterior disclusion.

(Fig. 11–24). The more pronounced are the balancing side contacts and curve of Spee, the greater must be the thickness of the splint or the height of the cuspid rise or both. Minimize axial surface guidance. As is possible, guidance should occur between the tip of the cusp and the cusp ridge; however, the degree of balancing and protrusive interferences will alter this possibility. In effect, it may be necessary to guide on axial surfaces in lateral and protrusive movements because of an exaggerated curve of Spee or balancing side contact. The general principle is: *The greater the cuspid rise required, the more the axial surface will be needed to provide disclusion in lateral and lateral protrusive.* Thus the thickness of the splint (its vertical dimension) and the height of the cuspid rise must be considered in the design of the splint to avoid excessive guidance (entrapment of mandibular

movement) on the axial surface of the mandibular cuspid. A general principle: *Increase the thickness of the splint rather than cuspid guidance height for temporomandibular joint–muscle pain dysfunction; increase the height of cuspid guidance and reduce the thickness of the splint for bruxism.*

PROCESSING

The maxillary cast with the wax splint is removed and processed in clear acrylic. When a splint is returned from a commercial laboratory, it may not be removed from the cast on which it was processed unless there were instructions otherwise. In our experience, the processed splint should be removed from the cast but the inner (tooth) surface should not be polished. Final adjustment and polishing of the splint should be left to the dentist. Occlusal stops and retention are easily lost with polishing.

The splint should be returned from the laboratory in a plastic bag containing water to which a small amount of preservative or detergent has been added.

The use of a split cast mounting may be of value if the mandibular cast has been mounted in centric relation.

INSERTION AND INITIAL ADJUSTMENT OF SPLINT

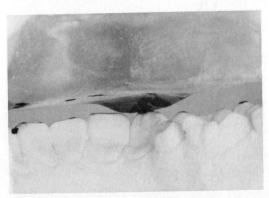

Figure 11–24. Waxing splint. Cuspid rise with ideal "fan" shape on hard inlay wax.

The processed splint should not be fitted onto a duplicate cast. It will not "snap" onto the teeth unless all major lingual undercuts were blocked out before waxing. On the other hand, it will rock in the mouth if buccal undercuts were blocked out or retention was removed in polishing. Because of the horseshoe design of the splint and dimensional changes in the acrylic after removal from the cast, the insertion of the splint may be difficult if careful attention was not paid to the blocking out of lingual undercuts.

Insertion

Because of the horseshoe shape of the splint, there is a possibility of causing the ends to be displaced outward slightly during the insertion provided that the lingual axial contours of molars and premolars have been blocked out adequately. This displacement allows the facial contours of the splint to pass over moderate undercuts and facial contours of the teeth. The least outward deflection will occur at the canine area. If embrasures, deep developmental grooves, and all lingual undercuts have been removed, only a few minutes are required to seat the splint. Grinding out the inner aspects of occlusal surfaces of the splint and using quick-cure acrylic to seat the splint is not a substitute for careful planning. A splint without retention or one that "rocks" should be redone.

Initial Adjustment

The splint must be adjusted at the initial appointment as well as at the time of subsequent appointments. Since contact relations at the increased vertical of the splint, especially with temporomandibular joint problems, may be different from those at centric occlusion, centric relation, or some other vertical, some adjustment of the surface of the splint is almost always necessary.

Objectives. Besides delivery of the splint, the principal objective of the initial adjustment is to provide even bilateral and posterior contacts, remove any balancing and any incisal protrusive contacts, and make the splint comfortable relative to bulk, especially lingual to the incisors and along the lip line. The splint should have a feather edge on the palatal side, and the periphery should not cross over rugae. The incisive papilla should have been given relief at the time of the block-out procedure.

Insertion Complaint. At insertion of the splint make certain that it is fully seated and the patient has no complaints, especially regarding "pressure on the incisors." If pressure is felt, it can be eliminated by careful internal grinding with a small bur (No. ½ round). Usually the embrasure areas that have not been adequately blocked cause the complaint. If sharp or ragged edges on facets of incisal wear were not brushed with stone at the time of the block-out, the areas may have to be adjusted if pressure on the incisors exists. Do not let the patient dictate the adjustment procedure.

In some instances the loose tissue of the cheek may become trapped between the splint and the teeth. This can be avoided by careful insertion of the appliance rather than removal of retentive areas on the splint.

Adjustment Procedure Steps

1. Have the patient tap lightly into splint centric. Use articulating paper* or ribbon to mark contacts. Adjust until bilateral/anterior/posterior contacts in centric are present.
2. Guide the patient into centric relation (if possible) or into a more retrusive position than tapping centric and mark contacts. There should be no slide from the retruded position to tapping centric when adjustment of the splint is completed for that day.
3. Guide the patient into lateral and pro-

---

*Premium thin (Mynol), Broomall, PA, 19008.

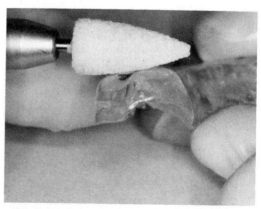

Figure 11–25. Adjustment of splint. All balancing, working, and protrusive interference must be removed.

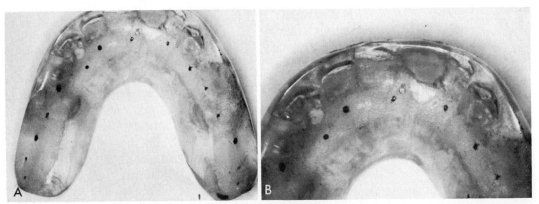

Figure 11–26. Splint contacts. *A*, even contacts bilaterally and A/P should be present. *B*, contacts should be small and be present for "tapping centric" and centric relation if possible.

trusive movements. There should be no working, balancing, or protrusive contacts away from splint centric except for cuspid guidance and approximately 0.5 mm freedom in centric. When interferences are present, remove with a fast-cut stone (Fig. 11–25).

4. After the splint is polished with pumice and Bendix, the centric stops should make very small contact marks (Fig. 11–26). The smoothness of the splint is a critical part of an effective occlusal bite plane splint. The splint should not have ripples and broad contacts. Bruxism and temporomandibular joint disturbances are aggravated when there are even minor surface irregularities present on the splint.

POSTINSERTION THERAPY

Effective splint therapy depends on a correct diagnosis of the dysfunction, the proper design of the splint, and proper adjustment of the splint initially and at subsequent appointments.

The design of the splint should not act to trigger bruxism. A splint may control bruxism and wearing down of the teeth in some instances; in other situations only the wear can be controlled because of the strong psychological factors that are present. Behavorial modification by biofeedback methods may be of added benefit. Psychological counseling may also be beneficial.

Adjustment of Splint

The splint should be adjusted in the presence of acute symptoms every five to seven days or less if the adjustment significantly influences the severity of the symptoms.

Differential Adjustment. In the presence of temporomandibular joint–muscle pain on one side, a patient will favor that side over the other and marking of the splint may be misinterpreted. Such protection of a favored side will cause articulating paper marks to be lighter on that side. Thus the operator should not attempt to obtain markings that appear to be equal in force bilaterally.

Adjustment for Swallowing. In the presence of pain, differential adjustment may have to be made for swallowing; oth-

erwise contacts should demonstrate even forces bilaterally on the splint. To begin, 28 gauge sheet wax is placed on the polished occlusal surface of the splint and the patient is instructed to make light contact with the splint. At that time the patient is asked to swallow. Contacts should be equally distributed. It may be necessary to use a water swallow. Patients may brace anywhere on the splint to swallow, so it is important that they "key" in on splint centric before initiating the swallowing reflex.

Maintenance Therapy

Under periodic supervision the occlusal bite plane splint may be used for long periods of time. Because it contributes to occlusal stability, the full coverage splint has been called a stabilization splint. Because some forms of temporomandibular joint arthritis are chronic and refractory to complete resolution, long-term splint therapy with splint adjustment on a periodic basis is necessary for control of discomfort. Such therapy is also preventive in nature inasmuch as the severity and number of exacerbations may be decreased by maintenance splint therapy.

Discontinuation of Therapy

Long-Term Therapy. Periodic assessment (6 to 12 months) should be made for possible discontinuation of long-term splint therapy. In some instances a trial period without the splint is indicated. Careful control of a patient with aggressive bruxism is mandatory. A new splint or other forms of therapy may be indicated.

Short-Term Therapy. A five to seven day schedule for an adjustment of the splint for acute dysfunction is seldom required beyond six to eight weeks. However, daily control of splint therapy may be required for severe functional disturbances.

SPLINT THERAPY AND OTHER THERAPY

The various aspects of splint therapy can only be briefly described here. The therapy varies for bruxism, temporomandibular joint–muscle pain dysfunction, phantom bite, diagnostic splint, chronic subluxation, temporomandibular joint crepitus and noise, acute and chronic temporomandibular joint arthritis, and restricted jaw opening. Differences in treatment are often based on symptomatology, the function that is disturbed, and the influence of treatment.

Splint and Occlusal Adjustment Therapy

It is often necessary to couple occlusal adjustment therapy with splint therapy in the presence of occlusal interferences that are obviously causing occlusal dysfunction.

Gross occlusal interferences should be eliminated before splint therapy is begun. Control of pain and adjustment of third molars may be necessary before extraction of third molars or before use of a splint.

Splint and Orthodontic Therapy

After initial splint therapy and reduction of symptoms, continued progress in eliminating discomfort may require occlusal therapy, including occlusal adjustment and comprehensive or palliative orthodontics. However, other than interceptive occlusal adjustment, comprehensive orthodontics procedures should not be introduced until symptoms have been brought under control.

If the temporomandibular joint–muscle pain dysfunction began during or following orthodontic therapy in which a stable occlusion could not be or was not obtained, palliative orthodontics may be necessary if the occlusal problem cannot be solved with an occlusal adjustment and splint therapy. Long-term continual splint therapy is not a substitute for occlusal instability that can be controlled by orthodontics. However, in some instances the lateral

discrepancy between centric relation and centric occlusion is too great to be corrected by even orthognathic surgery and long-term palliative occlusal therapy may be required.

In some instances it may be necessary to suspend active orthodontic therapy so that splint therapy may be used. The therapy can be done without de-banding provided that the appliance is passive.

Splint Therapy and Restorative Dentistry

The most common use of the splint in comprehensive restorative procedures relates to obtaining an acceptable centric relation registration for mounting casts on an articulator. The use of a splint to determine if an increased vertical dimension is practical in a full mouth rehabilitation is not recommended. However, it is significant if splint therapy does influence temporomandibular joint–muscle pain dysfunction in the presence of an apparent loss of contact vertical dimension.

DIAGNOSTIC SPLINT

A splint may be useful to determine if a reversible type of occlusal therapy will influence the symptoms of dysfunction. A provisional diagnosis and treatment plan should be reached as soon as possible and the splint should not be used for such purposes for longer than six to eight weeks.

Some individuals with real or apparent temporomandibular joint–muscle pain dysfunction have dependent tendencies or may develop these. The requirement of these patients for attention or treatment is unrelated to the presence or severity of symptoms. Psychological consultation before termination of therapy may be necessary.

Unit 11 Exercises

1. An occlusal bite plane splint is a _____ type splint used to

   treat _____ disturbances. A mouth guard is used in contact sports

   to control injury, especially to the lips. It is made of (soft, hard, pliable) material.

2. The major goal for an occlusal bite plane splint is to _____

   _____.

3. List three requirements for minimizing disturbing influences to the masticatory system:

   a. _____

   b. _____

   c. _____

4. Give the five highest priorities for physical requirements of a splint.

   a. _____

   b. _____

   c. _____

   d. _____

   e. _____

5. What is the general rule relative to incisal guidance?

   _____

6. List the main reasons for using a splint.

   _____

7. An exaggerated curve of Spee tends to require an increase

   in _____ of the splint and/or increase

   in _____ _____ .

8. What are the positions for mounting the mandibular cast?

   _____

9. Where is retention for the splint obtained?

   _____

10. What is the principal use of differential adjustment of a splint?

    _____

Unit 11 Test

1. The principal goal of occlusal bite plane splint therapy is to:

    a. cure bruxism
    b. prevent pressure on the joints
    c. protect the teeth from wearing down
    d. isolate occlusal contacts from the masticatory system
    e. stabilize the occlusion

2. What disturbing influences may arise from a poorly designed splint?

    a. interference with lip seal
    b. interference with swallowing
    c. a and b
    d. unstable splint centric
    e. a, b, and d

3. The device discussed in this unit is:

    a. a stabilization type of splint
    b. a mouth guard
    c. a and b
    d. not usable for longer than six to eight weeks
    e. a, b, and d

4. In the preparation of the cast for waxing the occlusal bite plane splint:

    a. block out all palatal side undercuts
    b. block out all embrasures
    c. a and b
    d. block out all palatal rugae
    e. a, b, and d

5. Which of the following general rules should be followed?

    a. open the vertical at least 3 to 4 mm
    b. place the cuspid guidance posterior to the mandibular cuspids
    c. have no incisal guidance
    d. have anterior occlusal contacts slightly heavier
    e. all of the above

6. The physical requirements of a splint are:

    a. full coverage of maxillary teeth
    b. "freedom in centric"
    c. cuspid guidance
    d. no incisal guidance
    e. all of the above

7. The preferred splint material is:

    a. chrome cobalt
    b. acrylic
    c. silicone
    d. rubber
    e. gold

8. A splint is adjusted for occlusal contact relations principally to:

    a. eliminate any unstable relations
    b. reduce vertical dimension
    c. reduce occlusal forces on teeth
    d. have contact of all supporting cusps
    e. reduce occlusal forces

9. Shifting of the mandible on a splint may occur in horizontal and vertical directions during a decrease of temporomandibular joint–muscle pain dysfunction. In the presence of pain on one side it may be necessary to:

    a. take all teeth out of contact on the painful side
    b. eliminate all posterior contacts
    c. do a differential adjustment
    d. raise the vertical dimension of the splint
    e. use a soft mouth guard

10. If all posterior splint contacts are eliminated and only the anterior teeth make contact on a splint:

    a. the posterior teeth may extrude
    b. temporomandibular joint–muscle pain symptoms may subside
    c. a and b
    d. the anterior teeth may be intruded
    e. a, b, and d

Unit 12

Waxing Functional Occlusion–2

In Unit 10 the wax-added technique was introduced as a means of developing a functional occlusion for cast restorations. Also in that unit the need was demonstrated for an occlusal adjustment to eliminate occlusal interferences in order to develop freedom in centric. In this unit the wax-added technique will be extended to include freedom in centric as a part of functional occlusion.

INTRODUCTION: UNIT OBJECTIVES AND READING

The wax-added technique for freedom in centric will be described; its value in diagnostic functional waxing will be considered. The principles for waxing the occlusal surfaces of a three-unit bridge are applicable to the waxing of restorations on dies mounted in working casts.

A. Objectives
1. Be able to analyze occlusal relationships for optimal placement of supporting cusps and centric stops.
2. Be able to describe the proper relationship between supporting cusps and marginal ridges, and how such relationships can be established by occlusal adjustment and functional waxing of a restoration.
3. Be able to discuss the step-by-step procedure of waxing according to the wax-added technique and the rationale for each step.
4. Be able to perform diagnostic functional waxing on mounted casts:
    a. based on an analysis of factors that determine occlusal morphology

    b. with prescribed wax-added technique
    c. to be compatible with functional criteria relating to:
        1. freedom in centric
        2. maintenance of contact vertical dimension
        3. proximal and axial contours related to functional occlusion
        4. freedom from all interferences to lateral and protrusive movements.
B. Reading (optional)
    Schuyler, C. H.: Factors in occlusion applicable to restorative dentistry. J. Prosthet. Dent. 3:722, 1953.

PREPARATION FOR WAXING

Materials

1. Study casts with lower first molar absent or cut away (Fig. 12–1A).
2. Hanau H2–PR articulator or equivalent.
3. Schuyler long centric pin and table.
4. Waxes:
    Ivory, inlay wax (hard, stick form). Inlay wax (hard) or Slaycris. (The hardness of the wax depends on room temperature.) Kerr 28 gauge casting wax (sheet form).
5. Instruments:
    Wax spatula No. 7
    P. K. Thomas Nos. 1 and 3
    Carver, fiber handle "C", S.S.W.
    Carver, Wesco 5C.
6. Quick-cure acrylic for forming pontic

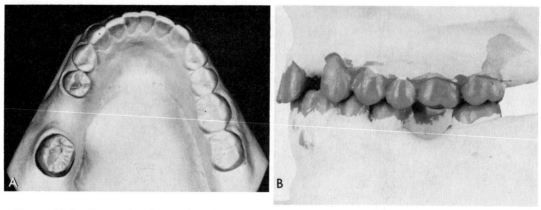

Figure 12–1. Preparation for waxing. A, casts with edentulous space; B, casts with occlusal surfaces painted with die-spacer.

(also to customize the incisal guidance if necessary).

Steps in Waxing

The first step is to paint the occlusal surfaces (Fig. 12–1B) with die spacer.* Next the casts or models are mounted in simulated centric relation. Then an occlusal adjustment to freedom in centric is completed. Next the incisal guidance has to be set. The abutment teeth for a three-unit bridge are then prepared, and the optimal positions for supporting cusps and centric stops are determined.

Mounting of Casts

In the clinical situation the patient has had an occlusal adjustment before the impressions for casts are taken, and a centric relation check bite is used to mount the casts in centric relation on the articulator. In the laboratory teaching situation the casts are mounted in a *simulated* centric relation (Unit 7, p. 114).

Set the condylar inclination to zero, the incisal guide to zero, and the incisal pin at the center of the table. Mount the maxillary cast centered vertically and anteroposteriorly. Incline the occlusal plane of the cast 10° to 15°. The maxillary cast can be mounted using a face bow. Move the condylar stop counterclockwise 1 mm. The

incisal pin is adjusted to contact the center of the incisal table. Mount the mandibular cast in maximum intercuspation with condylar inclination set at 25°. Reset the condylar stop back clockwise to zero.

Occlusal Adjustment

Make the occlusal adjustment to freedom in centric as discussed in Unit 9 of this manual. At the completion of the adjustment the vertical dimension at centric relation should be the same as that at centric occlusion (the pin in contact with the table at centric relation and centric occlusion and between).

Incisal Guidance

Adjust the long centric (FC) pin, the inclination of the incisal table (and lateral wings), and the offset pin as described in Unit 3, p. 50, so that there is 1 mm anteroposterior freedom in centric. The extent of the lateral component of freedom in centric is determined by the occlusal adjustment. The Schuyler pin and table may require customizing to provide full guidance for freedom in centric.

Preparation of Abutment Teeth

When a mandibular first molar has been lost and a second molar is present, a bridge from the second premolar to the second molar is constructed to replace the missing molar. The mesial abutment for the bridge may involve a full or a three-quarter crown and the distal abutment a full crown. The

---

*W/G 1-in-3, Sealer, Hardener, Spacer, Williams Dental Instruments, 520 Wildwood, Park Forest, IL 60466. Die-Spacer, Protex-M, 735 Ocean Ave., Brooklyn, NY, 11226.

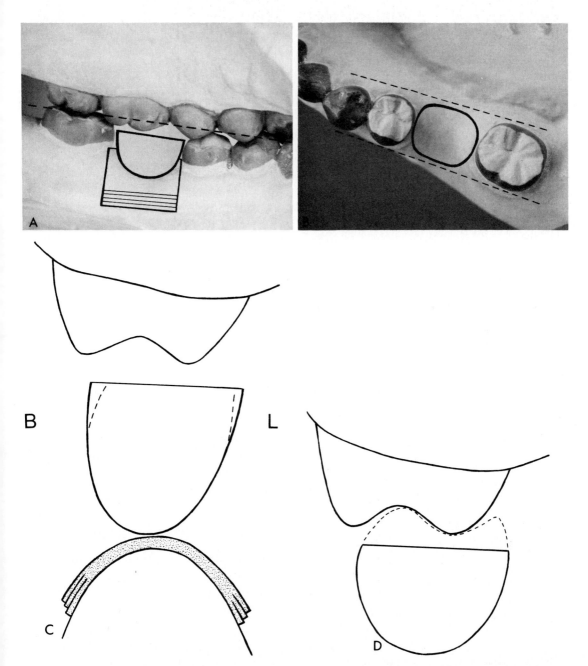

Figure 12–2. Preparation for waxing. *A,* positioning of acrylic pontic; *B,* buccal lingual position of pontic; *C,* pontic set on three layers of wax and trimmed along dotted line to allow proper waxing of axial contours. *D,* addition of wax (B = buccal, L = lingual).

reduction of the abutment teeth should be related to the replacement of the space with a pontic.

Prior to reducing the occlusal surfaces, mark the position of the supporting cusps on the occlusal surfaces of the maxillary teeth.

Reduce the occlusal surfaces of the teeth with a cross-cut fissure bur, green stone, or a sharp knife. Reduce the surface so that there is approximately 2 mm clearance between the cusps and fossae for all measurement. The amount of reduction is four thicknesses of 28 gauge green sheet wax. The general morphological features should be maintained. Bevel the buccal axial surface of the premolar so that the margin of the restoration is not a contact in centric or lateral movement.

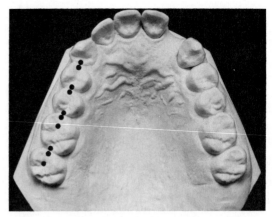

Figure 12–3. Preparation for waxing. Position of centric stops.

Pontic

Mold some quick-cure acrylic (dough-mix) into the form of a pontic. When set, the acrylic will be trimmed to the correct height and form for the position. Place three thicknesses of 28 gauge green sheet wax over the edentulous ridge area to prevent contact of the pontic with the tissues.

The pontic is positioned in relation to the occlusion of the opposing teeth and the position of the abutment teeth (Fig. 12–2A,B). Trim the pontic on the lingual and buccal aspects to allow proper contouring of the axial surfaces (Fig. 12–2C,D). The contours should conform to adjacent teeth. Seal the pontic in position and mark the postion of the supporting cusps.

Locating Cusps and Centric Stops

The first step in the development of a functional occlusion is an analysis of occlusal relations for optimal placement of supporting cusps and centric stops. Without considering the potential positions of supporting cusps in the planned restoration (the three-unit bridge) determine the positions for centric stops on the maxillary teeth for a "normal" occlusion. Whether or not the supporting cusps of the planned restoration should be or can be placed to match the centric stops as shown in Figure 12–3 depends upon the following factors: (1) occlusal stability, (2) freedom in centric, (3) working function, (4) avoidance of occlusal interferences, and (5) acceptable tooth morphology. The general principle to be followed is: *Place the supporting cusps in relation to the centric stops found in a normal occlusion — that is, if the arrangement of teeth is normal, interferences are not produced because of such placement and the likeness to normal tooth morphology is reasonable.*

Occlusal stability depends on a favorable interplay between all of the components of the masticatory system, not just the contact relations of the teeth. However, contact relations in centric relation, centric occlusion, and various excursions in both function and parafunction are important to occlusal stability. For cusp placement the principle of using a normal or near-normal arrangement of cusp to fossa and cusp to marginal ridge is based on conservation of tooth structure and on occlusal stability.

In relation to ridge and groove direction, the importance of knowing the pathways for cusps has already been suggested. The development of ridge and groove direction in the restoration and the accommodation for freedom in centric must be related to movements from centric occlusion and centric relation (Fig. 12–4). The line of triangular ridges and the direction of the developmental grooves should parallel or coincide with the paths of movement of the mandible in relation to supporting cusps. The presence of a freedom in centric, for example, 0.5 × 0.5 mm, suggests that functional grooves should be slightly wider.

The oblique ridge of the maxillary first

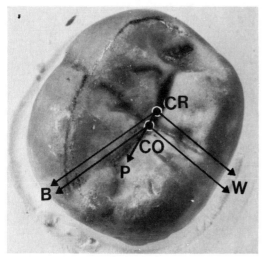

Figure 12–4. Movement patterns. *CR*, centric relation; *CO*, centric occlusion; *P*, protrusive; *B*, balancing, *W*, working.

molar (No. 3) should not be large. It should be low in height, distally placed, free from interference from the distal buccal cusp of the mandibular first molar (No. 30), and lie in the distal groove of the pontic or the lower first molar (Fig. 12–5). This groove must be slightly wider to accommodate freedom in centric and the path of the mesial lingual cusp of the maxillary first

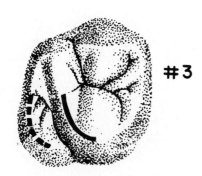

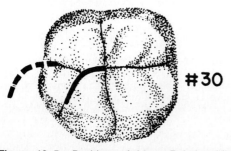

Figure 12–5. Positions of ridges. Relationship of oblique ridge of maxillary right first molar (no. 3) to distal buccal groove of mandibular right first molar (no. 30) in centric occlusion.

molar in balancing. The distal lingual cusp should be contoured to cross (dotted line) and contact the distal marginal ridge of the mandibular first (pontic) and the mesial marginal ridge of the second mandibular molar.

FUNCTIONAL WAXING

The waxing procedures follow a sequence so that supporting cusps can be placed in the most stable positions and occlusal parts may be added in relation to mandibular movements.

Step 1. *Placement of Supporting Cusps and Centric Stops*

Visualize the optimal position for the supporting cusps and mark with a pencil (Fig. 12–6). Freedom in centric from centric occlusion to centric relation was established in the occlusal adjustment in all areas except on the maxillary left first molar, the tooth opposite the edentulous space. The only area that will require an additional adjustment for freedom in centric is the central fossa of the maxillary first molar, because the supporting cusp of the second premolar and the mesial buccal cusps of the pontic and second molar occlude on opposing marginal ridges. With the development of the cusp cone that will contact the central fossa of No. 14 (maxillary left first molar), the oblique ridge distal to the proposed stop in the central fossa will have to be ground for freedom in centric relation.

Before proceeding to Step 2, make sure that there are pencil marks for each pro-

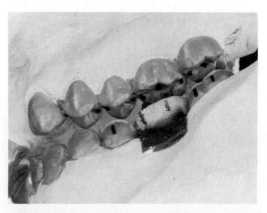

Figure 12–6. Waxing–step 1. Marking position of supporting cusps and centric stops.

posed cusp on the buccal surfaces of the mandibular prepared teeth to indicate where to start the wax cones. Be sure there are pencil marks on the maxillary teeth to indicate the areas for long centric or freedom in centric for each opposing cusp tip. Also, verify that the proposed centric stops are compatible with proposed pathways of movement, and that interferences are absent.

Step 2. *Develop the Supporting Cusps*

In centric occlusion, using the No. 1 PK waxing instrument, develop in Ivory wax* the supporting cusp cones in centric occlusion until occlusal contact is made (use zinc stearate to determine contact). Move the articulator into working, balancing, and protrusive positions and observe for undesired contacts (Fig. 12–7). Supporting cusps should make no contact in any position except in centric (centric occlusion, centric relation, and between) as shown in Figure 12–8*B*.

In *centric relation*, move the condylar stop to zero for simulated centric relation. From centric relation make lateral and

*Kerr Manufacturing Co., Romulus, MI 48174.

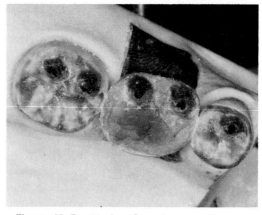

Figure 12–7. Waxing–Step 2. supporting cusps are tested with zinc stearate.

protrusive movements and observe for distortion of the wax. If interferences are present, consider placing the supporting cusp in another position.

Be sure of the following before going on to Step 3.
1. The incisal pin must contact the FC pin (test with shim stock) as the teeth contact in centric occlusion.
2. Each cusp cone must have a positive contact (tested by shim stock) in centric occlusion.

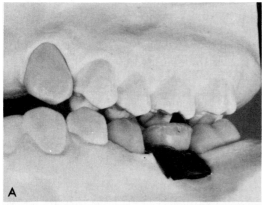

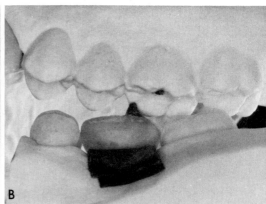

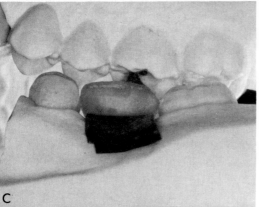

Figure 12–8. Movement patterns. Supporting cusps must not be occlusal interferences. *A*, relationship of distal buccal cusp cone to buccal groove of maxillary molar; *B*, relationship in balancing movement; *C*, relationship in protrusive.

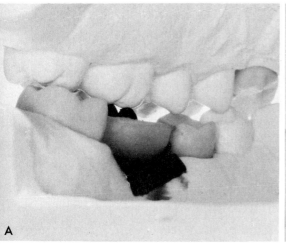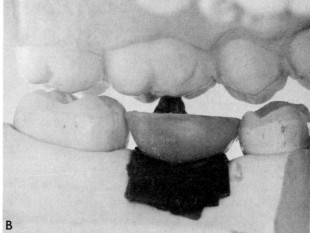

A   B

Figure 12–9. Waxing–Step 3. Centric stops on mandibular teeth. *A*, placement of stop for mesial lingual cusp of the maxillary molar; *B*, lingual view of position of stop.

3. The incisal pin must contact the FC pin in centric relation (test with shim stock).
4. There should be no posterior cusp cone contact in protrusive.
5. There should be no cusp cone contact in balancing.
6. There should be several contacts on the working side or if there is one contact it should be on the cuspid.

Step 3. *Develop Centric Stops for Maxillary Supporting Cusps*

The objective of Step 3 is to develop on the two abutment teeth and pontic the centric stops for the maxillary supporting cusps, i.e., the lingual cusps of the maxillary second premolar and the mesial and distal lingual cusps of the first and second molars.

Move the condylar stop into centric occlusion position. Verify the cusp tip (centric stop area) of each supporting cusp of the maxillary teeth and indicate with a pencil on the abutment teeth and pontic the proposed position of the centric stop for each maxillary supporting cusp. At this time develop centric stops only for the maxillary premolar and the mesial lingual cusps of the molars. The other stops will be developed when the marginal ridges are developed. Begin the development of the centric stop on the pontic by adding Ivory wax opposite the supporting cusp marked with the pencil (viz., mesial lingual cusp of No. 14). Keep adding wax

until contact is established (Fig. 12–9). While the wax is still molten, move the upper member of the articulator between centric occlusion and centric relation until the whole area between centric occlusion and centric relation is formed in wax into an area of freedom in centric (long centric). The height of the centric stop can be established by first using zinc stearate (Fig. 12–10) and then closing the articulator. Shim stock can be used also during the procedure. The entire centric occlusion–centric relation mark should be present.

Use zinc stearate to check the form of centric stop for stability. Figure 12–11 is a cross section (BL) of centric stops and supporting cusps showing stable and unstable relations. The stable stop is relatively flat except at margins where the

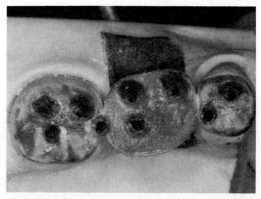

Figure 12–10. Contacts in centric. Check contacts in centric with zinc stearate.

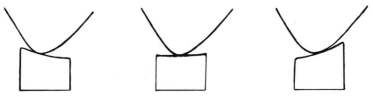

Figure 12–11. Form of centric stops. Cusp tips should not make contact on an incline. Cusp tip should make contact as shown in middle diagram.

buccal and lingual inclines of the cusps will meet the centric stop area.

Check for the following before proceeding to Step 4: Each supporting cusp cone contacts the waxed stop in centric occluson and centric relation (check with shim stock). The shape of the centric stop must produce a stable stop.

Step 4. *Develop the Nonsupporting Cusps*

The objective of Step 4 is the development of the nonsupporting cusps on the mandibular second premolar, pontic, and second molar (Fig. 12–12).

Move the upper member of the articulator into left working. The mandibular nonsupporting cusps must be placed so as to avoid the supporting cusps of the maxillary second premolar and the first and second molars. For example, the distal lingual cusp of the left maxillary first molar (No. 14) must not make contact with the lingual cusp cones that are to be developed on the pontic.

Mark the position of the mesial and distal lingual cusps of the abutment teeth and the pontic. The nonsupporting cusps of the left mandibular first molar (No. 19) should be placed: (1) mesially and distally

enough for the mesial lingual cusp of No. 14 to pass freely, and (2) lingually far enough to avoid the mesial slope of the triangular ridge of the distal lingual cusp of No. 14. The cusps should be high enough to prevent tongue biting. This can be assured by relating the cusp height to the adjacent teeth on the same side, the involved teeth prior to occlusal reduction or to teeth on the opposite side of the arch.

Develop the nonsupporting cusps of the proposed three-unit bridge using the green wax. There are six cusps to develop: a mesial and a distal cusp each on the second premolar, the pontic, and the second molar.

Before proceeding to Step 5 make sure of the following: The nonsupporting cusps should not interfere with lateral and protrusive movements. Also, the nonsupporting cusps should be relatively short and smaller and nearer to the lingual edge of the occlusal surface than the supporting cusps.

Step 5. *Develop the Cusp and Marginal Ridges and Axial Contours*

The objectives of Step 5 are to (1) develop the cusp and marginal ridges in such a way as to avoid developing occlusal inter-

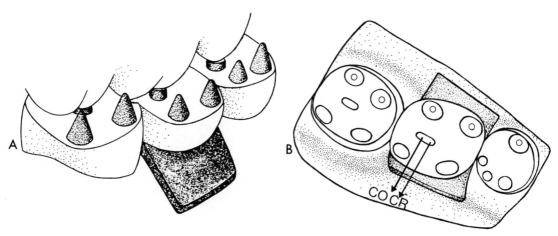

Figure 12–12. Waxing–Step 4. *A,* development of nonsupporting cusps; *B,* cusps should be placed to avoid contact in movements from CO and CR.

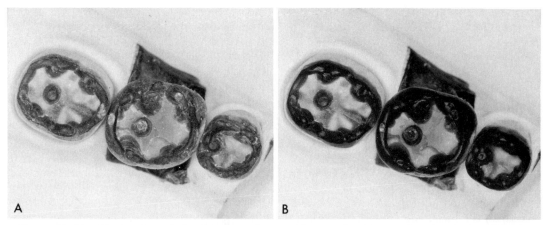

Figure 12–13. Waxing–Step 5. Development of cusp ridges and axial contours. *A,* use zinc stearate to determine centric stops and locate interferences; *B,* centric stops are maintained on marginal ridges.

ferences in mandibular movements, and (2) develop centric stops on marginal ridges for the distal lingual cusps of the maxillary first and second molars. Wax is added in small increments and dusted with zinc stearate (Fig. 12–13) and interfences to movements are tested.

Add green wax to the periphery of the occlusal surfaces of the mandibular teeth to form the cusp and marginal ridges and cavo (axial) surfaces (Fig. 12–14A,B,C). Do not carry wax onto the tips of cusp cones of the supporting or nonsupporting cusps. Leave the central portion of the occlusal

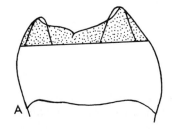

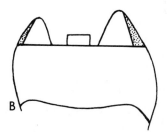

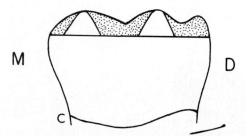

Figure 12–14. Waxing–Step 5. Wax is added beginning with the cusp tips and extending to axial surfaces and mesial and distal contact areas. *A,* marginal ridge; *B,* axial contour; and *C,* buccal surface. *M.* mesial, *D,* distal.

surface open as you develop the cusp and marginal ridges. Develop the centric stops for the distal lingual cusps of the maxillary teeth.

In forming the axial surfaces (cavosurfaces) do not overcontour because these surfaces are important to protection of the gingiva and to proper working contacts when indicated.

Be sure of all of the following before continuing to Step 6:

1. There are no posterior tooth parts that make contact in protrusive.
2. Only the cuspid and, where indicated, posterior teeth make contact in working movement either from centric occlusion, centric relation, or between.
3. No posterior tooth parts make contact in mandibular movements on the balancing side either from centric occlusion, centric relation, or between.
4. There should be a long centric stop from centric occlusion to centric relation for anteroposterior freedom in centric and a wide centric stop from centric occlusion to centric relation. There should be no interferences to closure into centric.

Step 6. *Develop Triangular Ridges and Grooves*

The objective of Step 6 is to develop triangular ridges and developmental grooves free of interferences in lateral and protrusive movements and with freedom in centric present (Fig. 12–15A,B).

Develop the triangular ridges by adding green wax but do not alter the height of the cusps, the position of the cusp tip, or the dimensions of freedom in centric (Fig. 12–16A,B). The triangular ridges (TR) are added a step at a time. Note that the centric stop (C) for freedom in centric has not changed once formed, and that the mesial lingual cusp (MLC) is widely separated from the distal lingual cusp. Also, the distal lingual cusp is quite distally placed and allows for the mesial lingual cusp of the maxillary molar to move here without interference in working. A cross section shown by the dotted line (X) demonstrates the buccal-lingual characteristics of freedom in centric (C). There is a gentle change between the occlusal faces of the triangular ridges and the freedom in centric stop. The ridge and groove direction should follow the direction of mandibular movement so as to minimize the possibility of developing interferences in the restorations.

Add a small amount of green wax to form a remaining occlusal surface not involved in function. Develop the grooves and carvings so that the occlusal surfaces resemble "normal" teeth (refer to dental anatomy). The adjacent tooth or a tooth on the opposite side of the same arch may also be used as a reference. Areas of the occlusal surface that have become flattened from contacts during movements and from carving can and should be rounded again. Heat the small tip of the No. 1 waxing instrument and quickly re-melt these flattened surfaces. Upon cooling, the surface will be round again. Be sure to add zinc stearate to this re-melted area and, check for free lateral movements — i.e., no interferences.

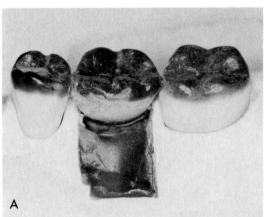 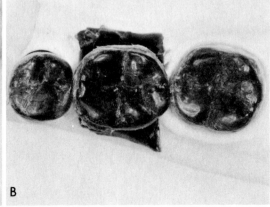

A   B

Figure 12–15. Waxing–Step 6. Development of ridges and grooves, *A*, view from buccal; *B*, view from occlusal. Centric stops must be maintained. Use zinc stearate for better observation.

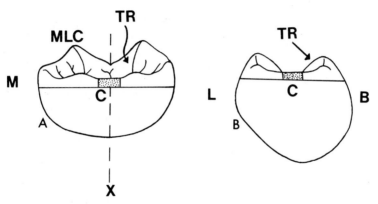

Figure 12–16. Waxing–Step 6. *A*, development of triangular ridges (TR) on mesial lingual cusp (MLC) and distal lingual cusp, *C*, centric stop; *L*, lingual; *B*, buccal. *C*, centric stop. *B*, view of pontic from X section.

Use the No. 3 waxing instrument and refine and burnish polish the grooves of the waxed occlusion. The waxed restoration (Fig. 12–17A,B) has yet to be refined and polished. Do not lose centric stops. Check with an instructor before completing the waxing any further. Some changes may be required.

Final waxing of grooves may be done at this time. Developmental grooves are formed between the cusp lobes to provide passageways for the supporting cusps from centric positions to lateral positions. Therefore, the angles of the grooves must be in relationship to the supporting cusps as they function around the condylar determinants. Make sure they are wide enough and deep enough to provide clearances for the cusp tips. Use the waxing instrument No. 3 to sharpen the groove.

Supplemental grooves are small grooves on either side of the triangular ridges dividing the occluding surfaces into a series of ridges that break up potential flat surfaces. These grooves minimize the total contact area of the occluding parts and also provide voids and wider grooves for better passageways. Chewing efficiency is related to areas of near contact as well as to areas of contact.

The wax-up is complete if all of the following are true:

1. The incisal pin still touches the long centric pin in centric relation and centric occlusion.
2. The supporting cusps contact the long centric stops in centric relation and centric occlusion (use zinc stearate).
3. All of the waxed parts clear in protrusive (use zinc stearate).
4. All of the waxed parts clear in balancing (use zinc stearate).
5. There should be contact in working on teeth other than the waxed teeth (the cuspid, at least).
6. The supporting cusps and the long centric stops are the only parts that contact in centric (use zinc stearate).

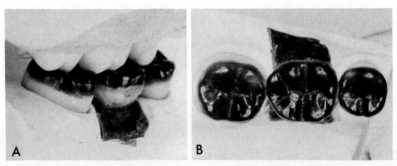

Figure 12–17. Waxing–Step 6. Polishing of all surfaces is done after working, balancing, and protrusive movements are made from centric occlusion and centric relation. *A*, view from lingual; *B*, occlusal view.

Unit 12 Exercises

1. What is occlusal stability?

   _____

   _____

2. What is freedom in centric?

   _____

3. Why are supporting cusps formed before nonsupporting cusps?

   _____

4. Can freedom of centric be incorporated in an individual restoration? (yes, no) If yes, when?

   _____

5. What is done in the clinical situation to unopposed posterior teeth in preparation for a bridge and waxing to freedom in centric?

   _____

6. Should the incisal pin make contact with the incisal table in the centric relation position? (yes, no) Why?

   _____

7. What parts should make contact in the working position?

   _____

   _____

8. What parts make contact in centric?

   _____

9. What is of particular help relative to supporting cusps in using the wax-added technique of waxing?

   _____

   _____

10. What determines the lateral dimension of freedom in centric?

    _____

Unit 12 Test

1. If casts are mounted in centric occlusion and a full crown is waxed in the centric occlusion position, and then the casts are re-mounted in centric relation, the closure of the casts in centric relation may result in:

   a. premature contact on teeth other than the waxed molar
   b. premature contact on the waxed molar
   c. a and b
   d. a lack of centric stops in centric relation when the cast crown is placed in the mouth
   e. a, b, and d

2. In waxing a full crown restoration of a mandibular first molar:

   a. centric occlusion position for the mesial lingual cusp of the maxillary first molar would be the central fossa
   b. centric relation position for the mesial lingual cusp of the maxillary first molar would be the mesial fossa
   c. a and b
   d. a place is made for centric relation contact distal to centric occlusion
   e. a and d

3. In a "normal occlusion" centric stop and supporting cusp relationships are:

   a. cusp fossa
   b. cusp fossa/cusp ridge
   c. cusp fossa/cusp embrasure
   d. cusp fossa/cusp fossa/cusp ridge
   e. none of the above

4. With "freedom in centric" a patient may move:

   a. from centric relation to centric occlusion without restriction
   b. from centric occlusion laterally for about 0.5 mm
   c. a and b
   d. into centric occlusion or centric relation from rest position without restriction
   e. a, b, and d

5. The extent of freedom in centric is determined by:

   a. amount of lateral slide before occlusal adjustment
   b. anteroposterior component of slide in centric
   c. a and b
   d. sharpness of cusp tips
   e. a, b, and d

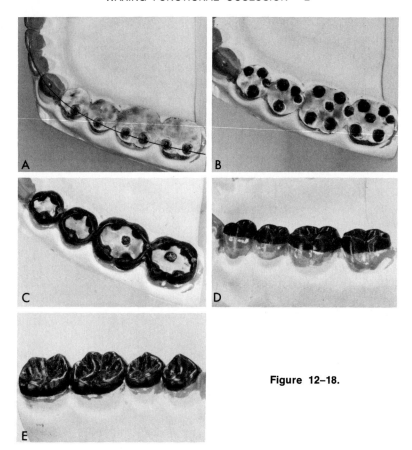

Figure 12–18.

6. In Figure 12–18A which waxing step is shown?

   a. step 1
   b. step 2
   c. step 3
   d. step 4
   e. step 5

7. In Figure 12–18B which waxing step is shown?

   a. step 2
   b. step 3
   c. step 4
   d. step 5
   e. step 6

8. In Figure 12–18C which waxing step is shown?

   a. step 2
   b. step 3
   c. step 4
   d. step 5
   e. step 6

9. In Figure 12–18D which waxing step is shown?

   a. step 2
   b. step 3
   c. step 4
   d. step 5
   e. step 6

10. In Figure 12–18E which waxing step is shown?

   a. step 2
   b. step 3
   c. step 4
   d. step 5
   e. step 6

11. In Figure 12–19 which waxing step is shown?

   a. step 3
   b. step 4
   c. step 5
   d. step 6
   e. step 7

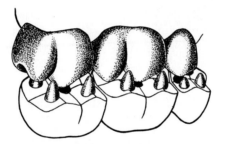

Figure 12–19.

12. Figure 12–20 is a view from above of Posselt's envelope of border movements. Indicate the area of freedom in centric.

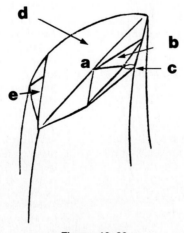

Figure 12–20.

ANSWERS TO EXERCISES AND TESTS

Unit 1: Exercises

1. changes during tooth eruption, tooth loss, increased mobility, etc.
2. contact vertical dimension
3. hinge axis; mount casts; centric relation
4. postural; vertical dimension; freeway or interocclusal; posterior teeth
5. balanced
6. imaginary plane; upper margin of the porion; lower margin of the orbitale; is not
7. condyle
8. physical (or mechanical); denture; natural; articulator; natural
9. arrangement; teeth
10. envelope
11. central fossa of the mandibular first molar
12. buccal

Unit 1: Test

1. d
2. a
3. c
4. a
5. a
6. a
7. e
8. c
9. e
10. e
11. d (sagittal plane)
12. c
13. a
14. b
15. c

Unit 2: Exercises

1. If increased table is elevated (increased from 0 to +1 or more), there will be an increase of vertical dimension and loss of occlusal contacts; may prevent protrusive excursion at extreme elevations
2. increase of vertical dimension
3. produce occlusal interference; loss of functional contacts
4. P–R adjustment; position of incisal pin
5. relationship between condylar shaft housing and condylar element
6. premature contacts in centric ("high" restorations in the mouth)
7. Restorations made for individuals who do not have an average intercondylar distance could have improper ridge and groove directions.
8. a. condylar slot
   b. condylar element
   c. condylar stop
   d. zero notch
   e. inclination indicating line
   f. spacer
   g. condylar guidance
   h. centric lock
   i. ear rod support pin
9. (1) pin not AP centered; (2) centric stops not set at zero for condylar elements
10. condylar element stop not set at zero on one side; condylar shaft housings not set equal on both sides.
11. (1) centric stops of condylar guidance not set at zero; (2) bent pin, incorrect condylar posts, manufacturing error; (3) incorrect length or positioning of incisal pin or height of incisal table
12. condylar element and axle not centered for all inclinations of the condylar guidance

Unit 2: Test

1. e
2. e
3. a (should be "lightly")
4. e
5. c
6. c
7. e
8. b
9. b
10. e

Unit 3: Exercises

1. incisal edges of the incisors, influence of condylar inclination, elevation of plane of occlusion, etc.
2. for disclusion of posterior teeth in protrusive and lateral protrusive movements
3. provide guide for waxing restorations and prevent wearing down of casts (maintain contact vertical dimension)
4. whenever the guidance cannot be set to allow all occlusal contact relations to be made
5. setting FC pin for contact in centric relation to centric occlusion
6. Freedom in centric is not present in the natural dentition unless an occlusal adjustment has been done and is reflected in the mounted casts. Hence, contact vertical dimension will not be the same at centric relation as at centric occlusion and the incisal pin will lose contact with the FC pin. Thus a flat long centric or freedom in centric would not be introduced into the waxing.
7. prior to taking impressions to make working casts, that is, casts on which restorations will be waxed
8. estimate freedom in centric in waxing
9. 1 mm
10. to the same extent as present in the mouth

ANSWERS TO EXERCISES AND TESTS

Unit 3: Test

1. a
2. c
3. e
4. c
5. c
6. e
7. e
8. b
9. e
10. c

Unit 4: Test

1. b
2. b
3. e
4. a
5. d
6. c
7. c
8. d
9. e
10. e

Unit 4: Exercises

1. no effect; at least ± 16 mm above center of notches on incisal pin
2. As the third point of reference is raised, the more shallow the horizontal condylar inclination will be when the protrusive record is used to set the articulator.
3. Error is approximately 0.2 mm on the balancing side if the incisal guidance is not changed.
4. the physical limitations of the articulator; that is, size of articulator
5. to avoid the possibility of an error as suggested in question 3
6. Simplify face bow transfer by supporting the posterior points of reference and automatically registering the arbitrary hinge axis.
7. yes, if the facebow is centered on the patient and on the articulator
8. 5–6 mm; ± 0.5 mm
9. a. to establish a third point of reference within the mechanical abilities of the articulator to handle casts
   b. to provide a reference for potential duplication of position of casts
   c. to provide meaningful relationship between the cast and the incisal and condylar guidance
   d. as a source of reference related to the angle of condylar guidance, plane of occlusion and angle of incisal guidance
10. no, some patients' jaws are noticeably asymmetrical
11. Casts may not be able to be articulated accurately in lateral movements because the condylar guidance prevents working contacts.
12. After mounting in the center of the articulator rather than in the correct position, tooth guidance can be increased by loosening the thumbnut on the maxillary cast and allowing contact to be made. Also, the condylar guidance may be changed to maximize contacts in lateral protrusive movements.

Unit 5: Exercises

1. an increase in contact vertical dimension
2. "high" in the mouth
3. is not
4. use full arch casts and do not use an interocclusal registration (wax check bite)
5. reduce axial contours of lingual cusps of maxillary molars and provide pathways for movement to cusp across cusp ridges of lingual cusps of maxillary molars
6. No, jaw positions, occlusal contact relations, and jaw movements are too complex to allow such precise preventive waxing.
7. errors in contact vertical dimension
8. Use a "large" articulator, also a functionally generated path technique, and a centric relation check bite. Such an approach is not always practical.
9. not always practical nor required
10. Relating cusp height to adjacent teeth. However, without the capability for lateral movements, it is impossible to precisely anticipate the proper contact relations.

Unit 5: Test

1. c
2. a
3. e
4. c
5. a
6. c
7. c
8. b
9. c
10. e

Unit 6: Exercises

1. a. absence of centric stops
   b. presence or absence of balancing side contacts
   c. presence of balancing side interferences
   d. presence of working side interferences

e. presence of protrusive interferences
f. position of CR contact
g. facets of wear and contacts in eccentric position
h. mobile teeth

2. aid in establishing whether or not mounting is adequate; possible problems that may prevent an adequate mounting of casts; aid in setting condylar guidance

3. mounting may not reflect occlusal relations in the patient because of functional disturbances; inadequate articulator; occlusion may change

4. Impressions may not reflect position of teeth at any given time and casts are fixed in position. For example, a centric occlusion position may not be possible if tooth is displaced by impression material.

5. working side interference

6. Yes, in a stable occlusion. Changes are likely to occur because of temporomandibular joint–muscle dysfunctions, habits, new restorations, orthodontics, etc.

7. a. It involves a new restoration.
   b. causes displacement of the tooth
   c. the tooth is in heavy function
   d. mobile because of periodontal disease

8. a. a change in the occlusion associated with periodontal disease
   b. temporomandibular joint–muscle dysfunction
   c. restorative dentistry

9. a. incorrect mounting of casts
   b. articulator not correctly adjusted or is inadequate
   c. error in impressions

10. Restorations may be made when occlusal relations are disturbed in the patient.

Unit 6: Test

1. e
2. c
3. a
4. e
5. d
6. e
7. e
8. c
9. e
10. e

Unit 7: Exercises

1. a. to compare the alikeness of contact relationships of the teeth on the articulator and in the patient
   b. to see what effect certain articulator settings have on the contact relationships of the teeth

2. a. clearance between posterior teeth decreases
   b. restored cuspal inclinations may be too steep, dictating posterior contacts (interferences) during protrusive excursions

3. a. clearance between molar teeth on the balancing side decreases
   b. no change
   c. In the patient there would be more clearance because the more shallow guidances dictates shorter, shallower cusps.

4. a. 1. distance between molars reduced
      2. distance between molars reduced
   b. 1. slight decrease in space between molars
      2. space between molars reduced

5. a. maxillary cast moves down and laterally to the right with decreases in space between shaft housing and condylar element
   b. shaft housing remains in contact with condylar element; thus, no Bennett movement occurs
   c. The resultant cusps may be too steep or tall; the lateral shift would dictate shorter, shallower cusps.
   d. Ridge and groove direction will be affected with possible interferences in lateral excursions.

6. a. Interferences (posterior contacts) may occur in the patient in protrusive and/or lateral excursions because of the more shallow guidances of the patient.

7. Condylar inclination should be 70 for the Hanau ear piece face bow; no support for the bite plane.

8. study purposes when patients are not involved; in the laboratory for class participation; for waxing a splint when centric relation cannot be obtained because of muscle hypertonicity; and when temporomandibular joint–muscle pain dysfunction prevents a centric relation registration

9. possible curvature of the condylar path; anterior and posterior separation of the casts from the wax check bite

10. condylar inclination setting more critical (difficult) than when the cuspid produces posterior disclusion

11. 25° for both simulated and actual CR check bite

12. The farther the condylar element and axis (axle) of the articulator are from the center of the condylar guidance, the greater is the influence on the position of the maxillary cast in centric occlusion as well as eccentric positions. It is necessary when maximizing tooth guidance to check for the right amount of contact in centric and eccentric positions. For example, make certain anterior and posterior stops are present for the condylar guidance that has been set.

ANSWERS TO EXERCISES AND TESTS

Unit 7: Test

1. a
2. b
3. a
4. d
5. c
6. c
7. a
8. b
9. c
10. e
11. e
12. c

Unit 8: Exercises

1. absence of centric stops in centric occlusion; casts come out of centric occlusion when thumbnut for upper member is tightened
2. balancing interference or condylar inclination or both not steep enough
3. point of attachment of Hanau face bow not on axis of articulator; only a third point reference assures that the maxillary cast is related to the axis of the articulator
4. anteroposterior error would be hypothetically zero
5. difference between that needed to assure some rocking movement with change of condylar inclination, and just enough to be in the area of straight condylar movement and within most functional range of condylar movement
6. functional disturbances; however, muscle hypertonicity and temporomandibular joint dysfunction usually prevent an accurate mounting of casts in centric relation
7. remount the casts in centric relation, check for errors in mounting procedures
8. inaccurate positioning of cusps and fossae in the centric relation positions; presence of premature contacts in centric relation
9. increased vertical dimension resulting in "high" restorations when placed in the mouth
10. None, if such working contacts are not present in the mouth. If working contacts are present in the mouth but absent on the articulated casts, waxing to occlusal contact on a restoration will result in a working interference on the restoration when placed in the mouth. If there are contacts on casts but none in the mouth, no interference or contact will be present when the restoration is placed in the mouth.

Unit 8: Test

1. a
2. e
3. e
4. b
5. a
6. e
7. c
8. d
9. e
10. c

Unit 9: Exercises

1. all have been accomplished
2. all of the above
3. smooth lateral movement of optimal working contacts
4. light or no contact is present on the balancing side and there are optimal contacts on the working side
5. optimal working side contacts
6. all of the answers
7. smooth gliding contact and the teeth do not move in protrusive movements
8. may require stabilization by new restorations
9. is not a problem without clinical evidence to support intervention
10. mesial lingual cusp of maxillary first molar

Unit 9: Test

1. d
2. d
3. c
4. e
5. b
6. e
7. e
8. b
9. b
10. d

Unit 10

p. 170 (1) a. indicate personal observations
b. avoiding the following and their effects on protrusive pathways: improper protrusive and anterior guidances, excessive cusp heights and angles, improper placement of anteroposterior grooves and positioning of ridges

ANSWERS TO EXERCISES AND TESTS

p. 171 (2) indicate personal observations
p. 171 (3) indicate personal observations
p. 171 (1) a. indicate personal observations
b. do not overwax triangular ridges;
provide reasonable axial contours; relate anatomical features
to those of adjacent teeth
c. indicate personal observations
p. 172 (2) a. indicate personal observations
b. provide for balancing pathways;
minimize mesial and distal cusp
ridges; do not overcontour axial
surfaces of lingual cusps
c. indicate personal observations
p. 173 (3) indicate personal observations
(4) (5) indicate personal observations
p. 174 (6) indicate personal observations
(2)   indicate personal observations
p. 175 (1) an occlusal adjustment to provide for
complete closure into centric rela-
tion and freedom to move from centric relation to centric occlusion;
also, the removal of working, balancing, and protrusive interferences
p. 175 (2) occlusal surfaces can be waxed without occlusal interferences being incorporated into them.

Unit 10: Exercises

2 and 4 (see Fig. 10–20)
3. slide in centric
5. a. on a plane–freedom in centric
b. at a point–point centric
6. the same as at centric occlusion
7. the same as at centric occlusion
8. premature contact in centric relation (occlusal interference to complete closure)
9. balancing and working interferences
10. occlusal interferences on the restorations

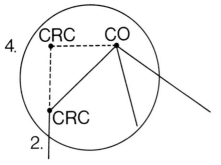

Figure 10–20

Unit 10: Test

1. e
2. c
3. c
4. d
5. a
6. d
7. d
8. c
9. b
10. c
11. b
12. b
13. c
14. c
15. a

Unit 11: Exercises

1. stabilization; functional; soft, pliable
2. isolate the contact relations of the teeth
from the masticatory system without introducing disturbing influences
3. provide for stable contact relations, allow
for lip seal if possible, do not interfere with
swallowing, others (see Unit 2, Goals for
Splint Therapy)
4. smooth, flat occlusal surfaces, freedom in
splint centric, cuspid guidance, no incisal
guidance, occlusal stability
5. no incisal guidance on splint
6. for treatment of temporomandibular joint–
muscle pain dysfunction and treatment of
bruxism
7. thickness; cuspid rise
8. centric relation; centric occlusion; or open
vertical
9. facial aspects–height of contour and interproximal areas of molars and premolars
10. to allow for slightly less contact force on
the painful side

Unit 11: Test

1. d
2. e
3. a
4. c
5. c
6. e
7. b
8. a
9. c
10. e

ANSWERS TO EXERCISES AND TESTS

Unit 12: Exercises

1. a state of homeostasis in which functional and structural changes are within the range of normal for the masticatory system
2. freedom of the mandible to close without interference into contact in centric occlusion, centric relation, and between
3. so that one can visualize and place this important cusp without having to see around the nonsupporting cusps
4. yes, provided an occlusal adjustment has been done first or one guesses at the dimensions
5. Usually the site of freedom in centric is established at the time of the occlusal adjustment.
6. yes, vertical dimension should be the same as at centric occlusion
7. cuspid/cuspid; mandibular supporting cusps and maxillary nonsupporting cusps; molars and premolars; at least the cuspids should make contact
8. only supporting cusps and centric stops
9. It is possible to exclude all parts of the waxing (restoration) from contact in lateral and protrusive movements yet maintain contact in centric.
10. the amount of freedom established during the occlusal adjustment or arbitrarily established in a full mouth reconstruction

Unit 12: Test

1. c
2. a
3. c
4. e
5. e
6. b
7. c
8. d
9. e
10. e
11. b
12. See Figure 12–21

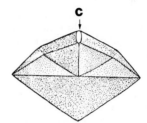

Figure 12–21

Index

Page numbers in *italics* indicate illustrations; page
numbers followed by the letter *t* refer to tables.